Glucose and Insulin Homeostasis

Edited by Alok Raghav and Rimma Shaginian

Published in London, United Kingdom

Glucose and Insulin Homeostasis
http://dx.doi.org/10.5772/intechopen.1000407
Edited by Alok Raghav and Rimma Shaginian

Contributors
Alok Raghav, Anchala Kumari, Anish Murtaja Alam Khan, Bandana Singh, Brijesh Kumar Mishra, Chelsea Giroir, Ebenezer Akinnusi, Enrique Valdés Rubio, Gausal A. Khan, Goo-Bo Jeong, Helen Calmes, Issa Rasheed Fetian, Kenan Sakar, Mohammed Eid Alqahtani, Mukesh Jain, Nese Cinar, Olorunfemi Oyewole Babalola, Opeyemi Iwaloye, Paul Olamide Ottu, Pinky Shukla, Precious Olayinka Aturamu, Swati Sharma, Venera Berisha-Muharremi

First published in London, United Kingdom, 2024 by IntechOpen
IntechOpen is the global imprint of INTECHOPEN LIMITED, registered in England and Wales, registration number: 11086078, 167-169 Great Portland Street, London, W1W 5PF, United Kingdom

British Library Cataloguing-in-Publication Data
A catalogue record for this book is available from the British Library

Additional hard and PDF copies can be obtained from orders@intechopen.com

Glucose and Insulin Homeostasis
Edited by Alok Raghav and Rimma Shaginian
p. cm.
Print ISBN 978-1-83769-932-2
Online ISBN 978-1-83769-931-5
eBook (PDF) ISBN 978-1-83769-933-9

For EU product safety concerns:
IN TECH d.o.o., Prolaz Marije Krucifikse Kozulić 3, 51000 Rijeka, Croatia,
info@intechopen.com or visit our website at intechopen.com.

Meet the editors

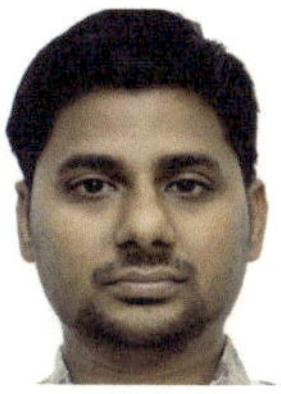

Dr. Alok Raghav obtained his Ph.D. in Endocrinology from Rajiv Gandhi Centre for Diabetes and Endocrinology, J.N. Medical College, Faculty of Medicine, Aligarh Muslim University, India. He worked as a project scientist at the Indian Institute of Technology in Kanpur, India. He has more than 10 years of research experience in glycobiology and diabetes mellitus. He also worked as Scientist C at the Multidisciplinary Research Unit (sponsored by the Department of Health Research, Ministry of Health and Family Welfare, New Delhi), GSVM Medical College Kanpur, India. He is currently a research professor at the School of Medicine, Department of Anatomy & Cell Biology, Lee Gil Ya Cancer and Diabetes Institute, Gachon University, South Korea. Dr. Raghav has received several international and national awards. He is also an associate editor for Frontiers in Endocrinology and Frontiers in Public Health and an academic editor for PLOS One.

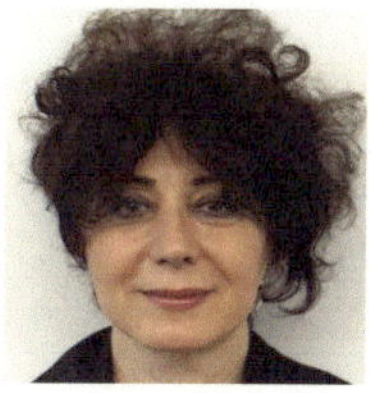

Rimma Shaginian, MD, specializes in diabetes endocrinology and cardiometabolic disorders. She has more than 10 years of clinical experience in clinical endocrinology, including diabetes, obesity, metabolic syndrome, cardiovascular endocrinology, growth hormone disorders, and bone metabolism disorders. She has more than 12 years of experience working in the pharmaceutical industry, namely as a Medical Leader of Diabetes at Eli Lilly. She also has more than 7 years of experience in the diabetes technology industry/Ascensia Diabetes care, leading the medical affairs team and conducting research to assess clinical aspects of blood glucose monitoring (BGM), continuous glucose monitoring (CGM), and diabetes digital applications. She is an author of more than forty original research papers, reviews, abstracts, and posters. She is a speaker at various diabetes training courses and several national and international congresses.

Contents

Preface

Glucose and Insulin Homeostasis is a collection of reviewed and relevant research chapters that discuss recent developments in endocrinology. It includes scholarly contributions from various authors edited by a group of experts in the field.

The book includes the following nine chapters:

Chapter 1: "Hypoglycemia in the Hospitalized Patient: Interventions and Opportunities"

Chapter 2: "Hypoglycemia in Type 1 Diabetes Mellitus"

Chapter 3: "Impact of the Use of Metformin in the Prevention of Gestational Diabetes Mellitus in the High-Risk Population: An Article Review"

Chapter 4: "Unveiling the Significance of the 'Bathtub' Shape in Blood Glucose Curve Analysis"

Chapter 5: "Estimation of HbA1c and Impact of Continuous Glucose Monitoring in Hypoglycemic States"

Chapter 6: "Perspective Chapter: Crosstalk between Bone Metabolism and Insulin Resistance"

Chapter 7: "Stress-Induced Insulin Resistance: Role of Von Willebrand Factor"

Chapter 8: "Lifestyle Interventions to Manage Insulin Resistance"

Chapter 9: "Exploring the Function of Inflammatory Routes in Insulin Resistance: Interpreting the Inflammatory Veil of Medusa"

The target audience is scholars and specialists in the field.

IntechOpen

Chapter 1

Hypoglycemia in the Hospitalized Patient: Interventions and Opportunities

Chelsea Giroir and Helen Calmes

Abstract

Hypoglycemia occurs frequently in hospitalized patients and can lead to cardiac arrhythmia/ischemia, seizures, or death. The Louisiana Hospital Improvement Innovation Network (HIIN) requires hospitals to report incidents of hypoglycemia as a quality measure. The purpose of this study is to evaluate the incidence of hypoglycemic events and identify precipitating factors at our institution. This is an IRB-approved single-center, retrospective chart review conducted from January to December of 2022 at an academic medical center. All admitted patients who received an antihyperglycemic agent and experienced a hypoglycemic event, defined as blood glucose <50 mg/dL (2.8 mmol/L), within 24 hours were included. The primary outcome assessed the incidence of hypoglycemic events. A total of 2455 patients received insulin during their admission, of which 91 (3.7%) had a hypoglycemic event that met inclusion criteria. Patients were predominately male (58%) with a median age of 53 years old. A diagnosis of Type I or Type II Diabetes Mellitus was reported in 73% of patients. Basal or basal-bolus insulin was ordered in 70.3% of patients. Our institution's yearly incidence of 3.7% is above the HIIN standard of 3%. Optimization of guidelines and order sets are proposed to help lower the incidence of hypoglycemic events.

Keywords: hypoglycemia, insulin, order entry, hospital, complications

1. Introduction

The occurrence of hypoglycemia, defined as a blood glucose reading of less than 70 mg/dL (3.9 mmol/L), in hospitalized patients has been associated with increased cost, length of stay, and most importantly, morbidity and mortality. Recently, data suggested that more than 25% of all inpatient days are incurred by people with diabetes [1]. Management of glucose proposes a challenge as patient-specific factors must be taken into account. For example, critically ill or elderly patients may not be treated as conservatively as a stable or younger patient would be treated [1]. The NICE-SUGAR trial showed that strict glycemic control can result in increased morbidity and mortality [2]. Other risk factors for developing hypoglycemia while inpatient can include severe comorbid diseases (sepsis, impaired renal function, malignancy, liver failure, and heart failure), other endocrine disorders, types and duration of diabetes, pregnancy, low body mass index, and improvement in patient's clinical status [3].

Symptomatic hypoglycemia is defined as a blood glucose level less than 70 mg/dL (3.9 mmol/L) accompanied by symptoms of hypoglycemia. Symptoms can include anxiety, irritability, dizziness, diaphoresis, pallor, tachycardia, headache, shakiness, and hunger. Symptoms such as malaise, lethargy, and slurred speech can occur due to effects on the central nervous system [4]. Because of this accredited organizations around the world, including the American Diabetes Association (ADA), all suggest that healthcare providers be notified when blood glucose levels are less than or equal to 70 mg/dL (3.9 mmol/L) [1] and should be the threshold to initiate treatment.

1.1 Treatment

According to the Endocrine Society Clinical Practice Guidelines, hypoglycemia can be classified into three separate levels [5]. The first level is defined as blood glucose 54–70 mg/dL (3.0–3.9 mmol/L). These patients may not experience symptoms and can ingest carbohydrates to prevent progression. If the patient is listed as 'nothing by mouth' (NPO) alternative sources may be given (I.e., dextrose 50% in water) Level two is defined as blood glucose less than 54 mg/dL (3.0 mmol/L), and places patient at an increased risk for cognitive dysfunction and mortality. Lastly, level three is classified as the occurrence of a severe event (altered mental status and/or physical status). These patients should be treated with glucagon or an alternative carbohydrate source [6].

Asymptomatic or symptomatic patients who are conscious, orientated, and can tolerate oral treatment should receive a rapid-acting carbohydrate. Examples of rapid-acting carbohydrates include 15–20 mg chewable glucose tablets or 150–200 ml of orange juice, and the effect should be seen within 20 minutes [7]. Blood glucose levels can be retested every 15–20 minutes, and if still less than 70 mg/dL (3.9 mmol/L), oral treatment can be repeated up to three times. For patients who are disoriented and/or unable to take it by mouth, 15 g of glucose gel, 1 mg of intramuscular glucagon, or 10 or 50% intravenous dextrose should be administered [7].

1.2 Financial impact

In addition to patient safety, the incidence of hypoglycemia also has an impact on cost. Between January 2007 and December 2011, hospital visits from Medicare beneficiaries, because of hypoglycemia, were more than $600 million in spending, and excess medical costs increased from $8417 to $9601 [8]. Studies have revealed that the cost to the hospital is $1161 direct costs per episode with a range of $242–$579 added for indirect costs: or non-medical interventions. No matter the severity of the hypoglycemic episodes, the economic burden remains. The short-term costs (e.g., emergency room visits) and the long-term costs (e.g., cardiovascular events, cognitive issues) contribute to the total treatment costs. One study by Curkendall, et al. set out to assess the clinical and economic impact of hypoglycemia that develops during hospitalization in patients who have diabetes. This study found that patients who experienced a hypoglycemic event had higher charges up to 38.9% [9]. The cost of the hospital is not the only thing that should be taken into consideration.

1.3 University Medical Center New Orleans

University Medical Center New Orleans (UMCNO) is a 446-bed non-profit, public, research, and academic hospital located in the central business district of New Orleans, Louisiana, providing tertiary care for the southern Louisiana region and beyond. UMCNO is one of the region's only university-level academic medical centers. UMCNO is also an ACS (American College of Surgeons) designated level-I trauma center. The hospital is operated by the LCMC (Louisiana Children's Medical Center) Health System, accredited by the Joint Commission (TJC), and is the largest hospital in the system. UMCNO is affiliated with numerous colleges of medicine and pharmacy. UMCNO is New Orleans' largest teaching hospital and training facility for many of the state's physicians. Meaning that our institution plays an integral role in shaping the future of healthcare for the region.

UMCNO's Post Graduate Year 1 (PGY1) pharmacy practice residency helps residents develop the necessary clinical pharmacy skills to help patients in their care. Part of this training includes involvement in patient safety and quality improvement initiatives. This includes training in Quality Reporting and Assessment Drug evaluation. Best practices are used to assess, improve, and make changes to medication practices at the hospital. Addressing hypoglycemia incidence at our institution is one such project.

1.4 Quality measure reporting

Adverse drug events (ADEs) in hospitals can be caused by medication errors, such as accidental overdoses providing a drug to the wrong patient, or adverse drug reactions [10]. ADEs place hospitalized patients at an increased risk of harm. Voluntary reporting and tracking of errors have served as the traditional method to detect ADEs. However, public health researchers have established that only 10–20% of errors are ever reported, and, of those, 90–95% cause no harm to patients [11]. Hypoglycemia has been identified as one of the top three preventable adverse drug reactions by the US Department of Health and Human Services [6].

The Hospital Improvement and Innovation Network (HIIN) was a national initiative from 2016 to 2022 that aimed to prevent patient harm due to adverse drug events and improve care in hospitals across the United States. The HIIN also served as precursors for the Centers for Medicare and Medicaid Services (CMS)-enacted guidelines. The HIIN had developed routine, required reporting by healthcare organizations on a statewide level for ADEs an injury resulting from the use of medication.

UMCNO has participated in the monitoring and reporting of the HIIN data for over 5 years. A benchmark of 3% or less of hypoglycemic events per 100 patients who received insulin was established. The equation used to calculate incidence can be found below.

$$Incidence(\%) = \frac{\begin{array}{c} Total\,number\,of\,hypoglycemic\,events\,in \\ patients\,receiving\,an\,antihyperglycemic\,agent \end{array}}{Total\,number\,of\,patients\,receiving\,an\,antihyperglycemic\,agent} \tag{1}$$

The HIIN requires patients who have a blood glucose level of less than 50 mg/dL (2.8 mmol/L).

Over the course of the last 3 years, numerous changes have been made to insulin order sets, admission orders, and diet insulin administration requirements for nursing staff. The benchmark at the target hospital has decreased from highs of 10 to 14% to the current range of 3–4%. The hospital should continue to implement changes that will further impact the hypoglycemia incidents; therefore, the purpose of this research is to define the yearly incidence of hypoglycemia at UMCNO and identify precipitating factors that may be contributing.

2. Methods

An Institutional Review Board-approved, single-centered, retrospective chart review was conducted at UMCNO from January to December 2022. Admitted adult patients, defined as at least 18 years of age, who received an antihyperglycemic agent were included. Antihyperglycemic agents included were insulin glargine, insulin regular, insulin lispro, and sulfonylureas. Patients were excluded if they did not have a hypoglycemic event (defined as blood glucose ≥50 mg/dL [2.8 mmol/L]), the event happened more than 24 hours after administration, or if the blood glucose recheck was ≥80 mg/dL (4.4 mmol/L) within 5 minutes of the original reading. A list was generated from the electronic medical record (EMR) of all patients who received an antihyperglycemic agent while admitted to UMCNO.

The primary outcome was to assess the annual incidence of hypoglycemic events at our institution during 2022. Secondary outcomes measured were patient-specific risk factors for hypoglycemia, insulin type ordered, dextrose administration, and documentation of symptomatic hypoglycemia. Symptomatic hypoglycemia was identified in the medical record through documentation within an hour of the hypoglycemic event occurring. Additional data points included baseline demographics, patient disposition, and mortality. This was a retrospective study and descriptive statistics were used to evaluate both primary and secondary endpoints. Therefore, no endpoints were calculated for statistical significance.

3. Results

There were 2451 patients who received an antihyperglycemic agent while admitted to UMCNO during the year 2022. After the application of exclusion criteria, 91 patients were eligible for analysis (**Figure 1**). Patients were predominately African American (n = 60, 65.9%) and male (n = 53, 58.2%) with a median age of 53 (interquartile range: 47–69.9) years old. A diagnosis of Type I or Type II Diabetes Mellitus was reported in 72.5% (n = 66) of patients. Incidence of hypoglycemia occurred most frequently on medical-surgical floors or units (n = 53, 58.2%). Most patients were discharged home (n = 47, 51.6%); however, 15.3% (n = 14) of patients died during admission, 26.4% (n = 24) were discharged to a medical facility (defined as either a rehabilitation, hospice, long-term acute care, or skilled nursing facility), and 6.7% (n = 6) left against medical advice (AMA) (**Table 1**).

The average yearly hypoglycemia incidence was 3.7% at UMCNO (incidence per month can be found in **Figure 2**). A total of 57.2% (n = 52) patients had a risk factor for hypoglycemia, including kidney/liver impairment (n = 26, 28.6%), sepsis (n = 9, 9.9%), or had multiple risk factors (n = 17, 18.6%) (**Table 1**). Symptomatic hypoglycemia was documented in 9.9% (n = 9) of patients. Basal or basal-bolus insulin was ordered in 70.3% (n = 63) of patients, bolus insulin in 23.1% (n = 22), 4.5% (n = 4) were initiated on an insulin drip, and 2.1% (n = 2) received a sulfonylurea (**Figure 3**). Insulin glargine was ordered through the institutional order set 23.8% (n = 15) of the time. Thirteen percent (n = 12) of hypoglycemic events occurred in patients receiving bolus insulin for hyperkalemia.

Home insulin regimens were restarted in 38.4% (n = 35) of patients, with only 65.7% (n = 23) of those regimens having a dose reduction. Patient education was documented in 25.2% (n = 23) of patients. A diet was ordered in 68.1% (n = 62) of patients, while 10.9% (n = 10) had no diet ordered, and 21% (n = 19) were "nothing

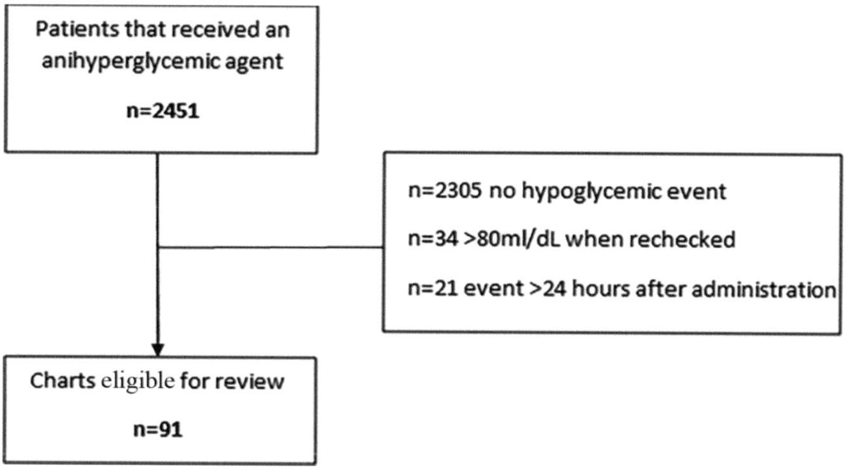

Figure 1.
Screening and inclusion.

Baseline characteristics (n = 91)	
Race, n (%)	
African American	60 (65.9)
White	22 (24.2)
Other	8 (8.8)
Asian	1 (1.1)
Gender, n (%)	
Male	53 (58.2)
Female	38 (41.8)
Median age (years) (IQR)	58 (47–69.5)
Median weight (kg) (IQR)	73.3 (66.9–86.1)
Type 1 or 2 diabetes mellitus, n (%)	
Type 1	12 (13.2)
Type 2	54 (59.3)
Not diabetic	25 (27.5)
Location of event, n (%)	
Floor	53 (58.2)
Medical intensive care unit	19 (20.9)
Surgical/Trauma intensive care unit	13 (14.3)
Other	6 (6.6)
Patient disposition, n (%)	
Home	47 (51.6)
Medical facility	24 (26.4)
Died	14 (15.4)
AMA	6 (6.6)
Risk factors, n (%)	
None	39 (42.9)
Liver/Kidney impairment	26 (28.6)
Sepsis	9 (9.9)
Multiple	17 (18.6)

Table 1.
Baseline characteristics including secondary endpoint of patient risk factors for hypoglycemia.

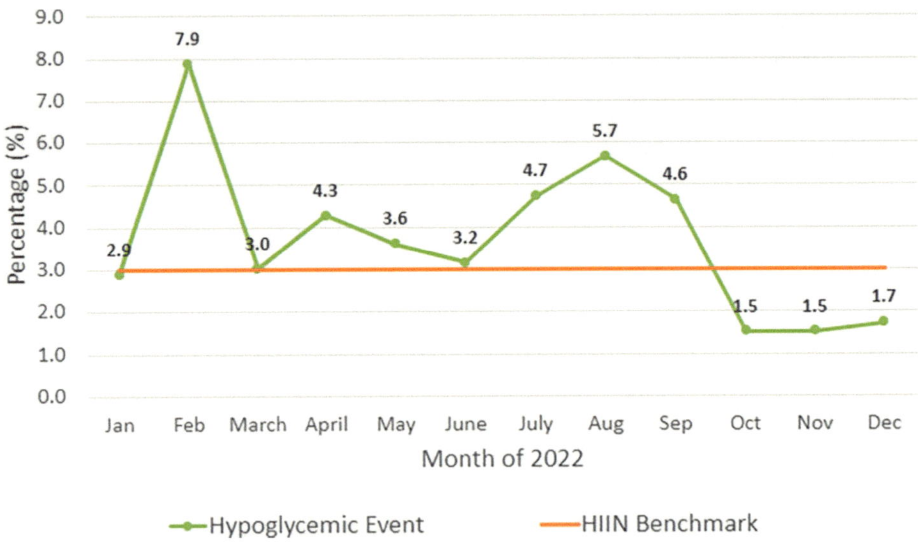

Figure 2.
Incidence of hypoglycemia; hypoglycemic events per 100 patients receiving an antihyperglycemic agent.

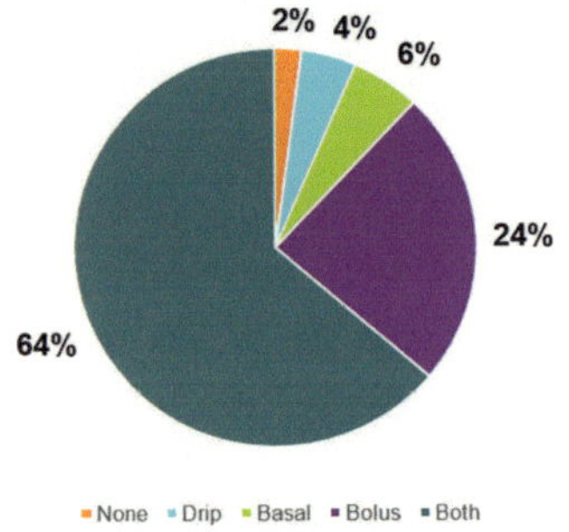

Figure 3.
Break down of insulin type ordered (n = 91). Basal-bolus includes basal corrective scale orders and/or scheduled insulin with meals. "None" includes the two patients who received sulfonylurea.

by mouth" (NPO). Dextrose was documented as administered to 41.8% (n = 38) of patients. Of the patients who were NPO, only 47.4% (n = 9) received dextrose.

4. Discussion

In this study, the incidence of hypoglycemia at University Medical Center New Orleans was 3.7% for the year 2022. The benchmark for hypoglycemic incidence for quality reporting is 3%. Hypoglycemic events lead to an increase in morbidity, mortality, length of stay, and cost [12], thus improvements in various areas must be made to decrease this incidence.

At our institution, clinical pharmacists evaluate every patient that is admitted to the hospital. Deferrals are implemented by our EMR system to assist the pharmacist in what needs to be addressed in monitoring including but not limited to patients' labs, anticoagulation, antibiotic regimens, and order optimizations (IV to PO interchange)

[13, 14]. Our institution currently has a deferral for hyperglycemia (**Figure 4**); however, previous studies have shown the implementation of best practice alerts (BPAs) and daily automated reports can decrease the incidence of hypoglycemia in the inpatient setting. Goldstein et al. conducted a study that implemented BPAs in patients who were deemed "at risk" for having a hypoglycemic episode. This study found that BPAs lowered hypoglycemia from 22.91 events/1000 patient days to 18.27 events/1000 patient days ($p < 0.001$). However severe hypoglycemia was not reduced [15].

After completion of the study, deferrals have been added to include a deferral for the pharmacist to review a patient's insulin regimen if there is a blood glucose reading ≤70 mg/dL (3.9 mmol/L). We identified that around 30% of patients did not have a diet ordered or were NPO at the time of the event; therefore, we also included a deferral for patients who were NPO or did not have a diet ordered while having an active order for insulin.

Originally, insulin glargine could be ordered without an order set through an individual drug order number (eRx). The eRx did not have administration instructions that were included in the order set, "DO NOT HOLD basal insulin when the patient is NPO unless MD is notified. CALL MD prior to administering scheduled basal insulin if BG prior to administration is less than 90 mg/dL (5.0 mmol/L)." Also ordering insulin glargine outside of the order set did not require point-of-care glucose checks to be obtained. To address this, the insulin glargine eRx was removed from the providers' list, allowing insulin glargine to only be ordered through the order set.

After the review of the order set was done, a forced stop was made so that a point-of-care test had to be selected (**Figure 5**). It was reported that home insulin regimens were restarted in 38.4% (n = 35) of patients, with only 65.7% (n = 23) of those regimens having a dose reduction. In our order set, there are areas of text space

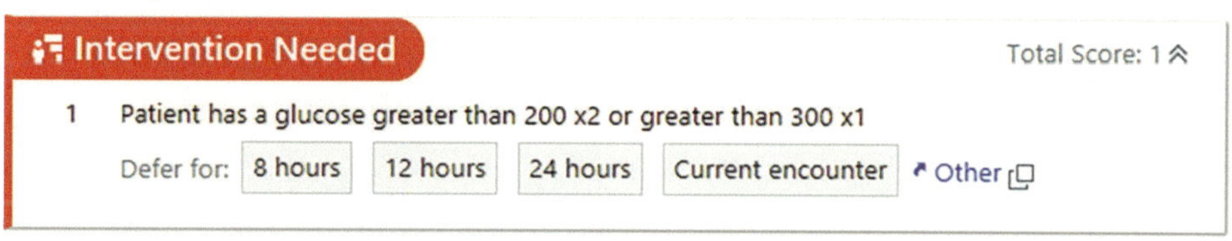

Figure 4.
Example of a pharmacist deferral for a patient who has had a glucose reading greater than 200 mg/dL (11.1 mmol/L) for 2 readings or 300 mg/dL (16.7 mmol/L) for one reading.

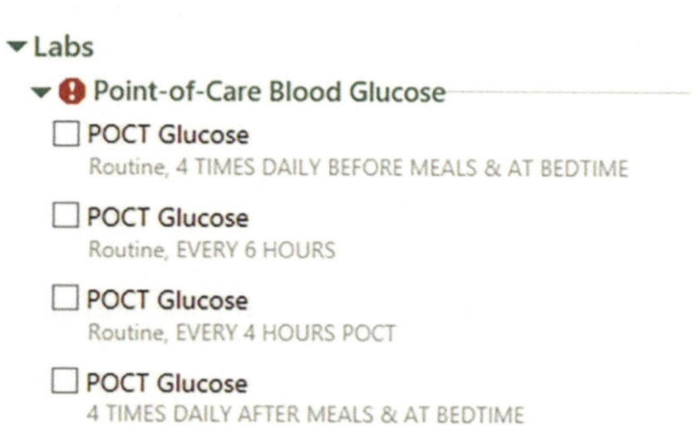
Labs
Point-of-Care Blood Glucose
POCT Glucose
Routine, 4 TIMES DAILY BEFORE MEALS & AT BEDTIME
POCT Glucose
Routine, EVERY 6 HOURS
POCT Glucose
Routine, EVERY 4 HOURS POCT
POCT Glucose
4 TIMES DAILY AFTER MEALS & AT BEDTIME

Figure 5.
The red stop sign with the exclamation mark allows the prescriber to know they will not be able to continue unless they select a point of care.

that can be utilized to help guide the provider to choose the right medication and/or dose. We decided to utilize function and add "If restarting home medication, consider a dose reduction by 25–52%."

Our study did not directly measure the costs of hypoglycemic incidents in the hospital setting. Accounting for and estimating costs attributed to diabetes and hypoglycemia is a health behavior that affects both the presence of diabetes and the presence of other comorbidities is difficult. However, we estimate that post-interventions the number of incidents will be lowered. Thus, the cost will be less.

While only 13% of events occurred in patients receiving insulin regularly for hyperkalemia treatment, a review of the hyperkalemia order set was also done. A study by Tran et al. looked to determine the frequency of iatrogenic hypoglycemia and develop an electronic order set to decrease the risk of hypoglycemia. This study identified lower pretreatment capillary blood glucose levels, previous history of hypoglycemic events, older age, lower body weight, and chronic kidney disease (CKD) as risk factors for hypoglycemia. They also found that about 92% of events occurred 3 hours after insulin administration [16]. Our previous hyperkalemia order set did not require a point of care to be taken after administration, only before. Therefore, we included an order for mandatory glucose checks before and 2 hours after administration.

One major limitation of this study is reliance on documentation in the patient's EMR for symptomatic hypoglycemia, if the patient received dextrose or patient-specific risk factors. Therefore, some of these could have been underreported in the study. Another limitation is that this is a single-centered retrospective chart review that could limit generalizability. While this was single-centered, the changes made to the order sets are implemented in other hospitals within the LCMC health system. This means that while our findings are institutional-specific, an impact will still be made with the changes implemented to help lower the incidence of hypoglycemia at other institutions.

5. Conclusion

The yearly hypoglycemia incidence of 3.7% is above the HIIN benchmark of 3%. Optimization to order sets has been established to lower this incidence. As mentioned previously, both the insulin and hyperkalemia order sets are system-wide. While the incidence of hypoglycemia is unknown for other hospitals in the system, changes implemented are likely to impact incidence at other institutions in the system as well. Provider and nursing education will also be established to minimize ordering and administration errors.

Acknowledgements

The authors would like to acknowledge Lillian Bellfi, Pharm.D., BCCCP for her assistance with this project.

Conflict of interest

The authors declare no conflict of interest.

Author details

Chelsea Giroir and Helen Calmes*
University Medical Center New Orleans, New Orleans, LA, United States

*Address all correspondence to: helen.calmes@lcmchealth.org

References

[1] Hulkower RD, Pollack RM, Zonszein J. Understanding hypoglycemia in hospitalized patients. Diabetes Management. 2014;**4**(2):165-176

[2] NICE-SUGAR Study Investigators, Finfer S, Liu B, et al. Hypoglycemia and risk of death in critically ill patients. The New England Journal of Medicine. 2012;**367**(12):1108-1118

[3] Pratiwi C, Mokoagow MI, Made Kshanti IA, Soewondo P. The risk factors of inpatient hypoglycemia: A systematic review. Heliyon. 2020;**6**(5):e03913

[4] Tomky D. Detection, prevention, and treatment of hypoglycemia in the hospital. Diabetes Spectrum: A Publication of the American Diabetes Association. 2005;**18**(1):39-44

[5] Seaquist ER, Anderson J, Childs B, et al. Hypoglycemia and diabetes: A report of a workgroup of the American Diabetes Association and the Endocrine Society. Diabetes Care. 2013;**36**(5):1384-1395

[6] McCall AL et al. Management of individuals with diabetes at high risk for hypoglycemia: An endocrine society clinical practice guideline. The Journal of Clinical Endocrinology & Metabolism. 2023;**108**(3):529-562

[7] Nakhleh A, Shehadeh N. Hypoglycemia in diabetes: An update on pathophysiology, treatment, and prevention. World Journal of Diabetes. 2021;**12**(12):2036-2049

[8] American Diabetes Association. Economic costs of diabetes in the US in 2017. Diabetes Care. 2018;**41**(5):917-928

[9] Curkendall SM, Natoli JL, Alexander CM, Nathanson BH, Haidar T, Dubois RW. Economic and clinical impact of inpatient diabetic hypoglycemia. Endocrine Practice. 2009;**15**(4):302-312

[10] Tsegaye D, Alem G, Tessema Z, Alebachew W. Medication administration errors and associated factors among nurses. International Journal of General Medicine. 2020;**13**:1621-1632

[11] Rozich JD, Haraden CR, Resar RK. Adverse drug event trigger tool: A practical methodology for measuring medication-related harm. Quality and Safety in Health Care. 2003;**12**:194-200

[12] Cruz P. Inpatient hypoglycemia: The challenge remains. Journal of Diabetes Science and Technology. 2020;**14**(3):560-566

[13] Destree L, Vercellino M, Armstrong N. Interventions to improve adherence to a hypoglycemia protocol. Diabetes Spectrum: A Publication of the American Diabetes Association. 2017;**30**(3):195-201

[14] Mathioudakis N, Jeun R, Godwin G, Perschke A, Yalamanchi S, Everett E, et al. Development and implementation of a subcutaneous insulin clinical decision support tool for hospitalized patients. Journal of Diabetes Science and Technology. 2019;**13**(3):522-532

[15] Goldstein R, Odom JM. 386-P: Inpatient hypoglycemic rate reduction through the implementation of prescriber targeted decision support tools. Diabetes. 2023;**72**(Supplement_1):386

[16] Tran AV, Rushakoff RJ, Prasad P, Murray SG, Monash B, Macmaster H. Decreasing hypoglycemia following insulin administration for inpatient hyperkalemia. Journal of Hospital Medicine. 2020;**15**(2):368-370

Chapter 2

Hypoglycemia in Type 1 Diabetes Mellitus

Kenan Sakar and Nese Cinar

Abstract

Hypoglycemia is a common problem in patients with type 1 diabetes and can be asymptomatic, mild, and severe. Despite therapeutic approaches and technological advances, hypoglycemia continues to be an important cause of morbidity and mortality in patients. Impairment in counterregulatory defense mechanisms and unawareness of hypoglycemia are the main risk factors for hypoglycemia. Recurrent episodes of hypoglycemia cause an awareness of hypoglycemia and defective counterregulation, resulting in hypoglycemia-associated autonomic deficiency (HAAF) syndrome. Efforts are needed to prevent hypoglycemia, and approaches include glucose monitoring, patient education, and medication adjustment. Advances in technology, such as insulin pumps and devices that allow continuous glucose monitoring, can significantly reduce the risk of hypoglycemia in patients when used appropriately.

Keywords: hypoglycemia, neuropathy, insulin pump, hypoglycemia unawareness, continuous glucose monitoring

1. Introduction

Type 1 diabetes mellitus (T1DM) is a disease that occurs as a result of the destruction of pancreatic beta-cells due to autoimmunity or different reasons and is characterized by absolute insulin deficiency and hyperglycemia. It is mostly prevalent in children between the ages of 7–15 and can also occur in adulthood. The fact that the disease can occur at any age and the annual rate of increase of 3% leads to a rise in the number of individuals with T1DM.

All individuals diagnosed with T1DM should undergo an intensive diabetes management regimen, which has emerged as the prevailing standard for the majority of patients. Intensive diabetes treatment involves the implementation of an insulin regimen closely mirroring physiological release patterns strategically integrated with lifestyle modifications, dietary considerations, and regular physical exercise. Vigilant blood sugar monitoring is strongly advised. Customized glycemic targets should be discerned individually, taking into account the dual objective of averting both macrovascular and microvascular complications, all while judiciously considering the potential risks associated with hypoglycemia.

Vigorous management of hyperglycemia holds significant significance, particularly in light of recent findings indicating an elevated risk of cardiovascular morbidity among individuals with elevated but still within normal range HbA1C values.

Consequently, the prevailing objective of care for individuals with diabetes is the achievement of normalized or near-normalized blood glucose levels. While lifestyle modifications retain their value in managing individuals with T1DM, it is imperative to acknowledge that optimal glycemic control is unattainable without the incorporation of insulin therapy. The administration of insulin, however, is not without its challenges, as iatrogenic hypoglycemia emerges as a complicating factor, posing limitations on the feasibility of achieving intensive glycemic control.

1.1 Epidemiology of type 1 diabetes mellitus

The incidence of T1DM shows variability across age groups, with a peak typically observed around 10–14 years. Nevertheless, T1DM can manifest at any age. According to recent studies, the global incidence of T1DM has risen over the past few decades, with an average annual increase of approximately 3–4%. In China and other Asian and South American countries, the annual incidence ranges from 1 to 3 per 100,000. Meanwhile, South European countries and the USA demonstrate rates of approximately 10–20 per 100,000. In Scandinavia, the incidence is higher, ranging from 30 to 60 per 100,000 [1, 2].

1.2 Pathophysiology of type 1 diabetes mellitus

T1DM is characterized by the persistent immune-mediated destruction of pancreatic beta-cells, resulting in a complete deficiency of insulin. The exact mechanisms triggering autoimmunity remain elusive; however, it is widely acknowledged that various environmental factors, within the context of genetic susceptibility, likely play a role. The destruction of beta-cells occurs at a variable pace and becomes clinically evident when at least 70% of beta-cells are either inactive or destroyed [3, 4]. The evolving risk of T1DM associated with migration underscores the significant influence of environmental factors in the pathogenesis of T1DM. This phenomenon has been observed in certain countries but not universally across all regions. Genetic susceptibility to T1DM is intricate, with approximately 40–50% of familial clustering attributed to polymorphisms in class II HLA genes encoding DQ and DR. The most high-risk haplotypes, DR3 and DR4, are present in 90–95% of young children with T1DM. However, less than 5% of individuals with HLA-conferred genetic susceptibility actually develop T1DM. Furthermore, there exists a diverse array of other genes that contribute to the overall risk. Children with a sibling affected by T1DM face a 5% probability of developing T1DM by the age of 20 years, compared to the 0.3% risk observed in the general population. Identical twins exhibit a 65% concordance rate when followed by 60 years of age. The risk for children of fathers with T1DM is higher (6%) than when the mother has T1DM, particularly if she gives birth before the age of 25 (4%), decreasing to 1% after that, akin to the general population. Remarkably, over 90% of individuals with T1DM have no discernible family history of the condition, although there might be a prevalence of other autoimmune diseases within the family, such as coeliac disease or autoimmune thyroid disease. The influence of genetic risk is more pronounced in individuals diagnosed at a young age and diminishes as the age of diagnosis increases. Conversely, patients with adolescent- and adult-onset T1DM exhibit lower twin concordance and decreased genetic risk scores [2, 5].

Childhood infections have demonstrated an association with an increased risk of islet autoimmunity and T1DM. In the TEDDY study, the incidence of respiratory infections and islet autoimmunity displayed a correlation in children under 4 years of age, reaching a peak between 6 and 9 months [6]. Enteroviruses, primarily, have been implicated as the predominant pathogens, and a meta-analysis revealed significant associations between infection and T1DM [7].

Moreover, some studies suggest that parental obesity, vitamin D deficiency, and dietary factors may increase the risk of T1DM [8–10]; however, the evidence is insufficient or weakly associated with the risk.

2. Hypoglycemia in type 1 diabetes

From a clinical perspective, hypoglycemia is categorized into mild or severe episodes. Mild occurrences of hypoglycemia do not induce alterations in mentation and can be readily rectified with straightforward measures. Conversely, severe hypoglycemia (SH) results in altered mental status, seizure, or coma and often requires external intervention (e.g., intravenous dextrose and glucagon injection).

In individuals with diabetes, pinpointing a precise plasma glucose concentration for diagnosing hypoglycemia poses a challenge, as the threshold for symptom onset varies among patients. Recurrent hypoglycemic episodes lower this threshold, while uncontrolled diabetes elevates it.

The contemporary classification of hypoglycemic episodes in diabetes encompasses three severity levels [11]:

Level 1 hypoglycemia is characterized by a plasma glucose concentration < 70 mg/dL but >54 mg/dL. The threshold concentration of 70 mg/dL is significant because it is below this level that neuroendocrine responses to hypoglycemia typically manifest in individuals without diabetes. In the context of individuals with diabetes, a significant number may exhibit compromised defense mechanisms against hypoglycemia or a lack of awareness regarding it. Consequently, plasma glucose concentrations below 70 mg/dL are deemed clinically significant in diabetes, mandating intervention irrespective of the severity of accompanying symptoms.

Level 2 hypoglycemia is characterized by a plasma glucose concentration below 54 mg/dL, necessitating immediate action to correct the hypoglycemia.

Level 3 hypoglycemia is characterized by a significant event characterized by alterations in mental status or a decline in the individual's physical capacity to perform tasks. This degree of hypoglycemia necessitates external intervention by another person to rectify the glucose concentration.

2.1 Clinical significance of hypoglycemia

Hypoglycemia poses a challenge to achieving optimal glycemic control in individuals with diabetes. Although the ADA Standards of Care [12] emphasize a patient-centered approach to glycemic targets, the overall recommendations lean toward rigorous, intensive glycemic control, aiming for an HbA1C level below 7% when the risk of hypoglycemia is low. This is due to the extensive literature [13] that tight glycemic control is associated with significantly reduced rates of microvascular complications. However, the goal of intensive control has also led to an increase in hypoglycemia rates, contributing to morbidity and mortality in certain patients [14]. Severe hypoglycemia is a common problem during intensive insulin therapy in patients with T1DM. The annual incidence of severe hypoglycemia among patients with type 1DM has been reported to range from 3.3 to 13.5% [15]. Severe hypoglycemia is reported to be the cause of death in 4–10% of the patients [16]. Because of the apprehension associated with acute hypoglycemia, individuals with diabetes might prioritize averting immediate risks over contemplating the long-term consequences of chronic hyperglycemia. Consequently, many diabetes patients may tolerate elevated glycemic levels as a strategy to prevent episodes of acute hypoglycemia.

The Diabetes Control and Complications Trial (DCCT) in 1997 revealed a substantial prevalence of severe hypoglycemia. Specifically, the incidence of hypoglycemia requiring treatment assistance was documented at 61.2 per 100 patient-years among individuals undergoing intensive treatment, compared to 18.7 per 100 patient-years in those subjected to conventional treatment [17]. Nevertheless, the incidence of severe hypoglycemia has exhibited a declining trend over time. An Italian study conducted in 29 diabetes centers during 2011–2012 reported a lower incidence of 7.7 per 100 patient-years [18]. Similar decreasing trends were observed in children and adolescents in Germany, Australia, and Japan [19, 20]. In contrast, the HAT study in 2016, which included 24 countries, showed a high incidence of hypoglycemia in T1DM patients. Rates of any, nocturnal and severe hypoglycemia were 73.3, 11.3, and 4.9 events/ patient-year for T1DM, respectively. The highest rates of hypoglycemia were observed in Latin America for T1DM [21]. Although advancements in treatment regimens may contribute to the decrease in severe hypoglycemia incidence, it remains a pertinent risk and ongoing threat for individuals with type 1 diabetes and their families.

Hypoglycemia may be associated with permanent brain damage and abnormalities in brain structure, particularly in young children with T1DM. Many studies conducted among children, adolescents, and older adults with T1DM have consistently demonstrated an association between severe hypoglycemia and a decline in cognitive function, particularly affecting tasks related to executive function and memory [22].

Hypoglycemia is associated with increased cardiovascular morbidity in patients with T2DM and T1DM [23]. The counter-regulatory release of epinephrine triggered by hypoglycemia increases heart rate and cardiac output. This response is also associated with hypokalemia, which has the potential to cause QT prolongation and other cardiac arrhythmias. Additionally, counter-regulatory hormones induce platelet coagulation and the release of proinflammatory cytokines, both of which impact vascular flow. When combined with the pre-existing vascular disease often observed in patients with diabetes, these factors create significant stress on the heart and contribute to cardiac morbidity.

Studies have shown that hypoglycemia is associated with an increased risk of fracture in patients with T1DM [24]. Compared to the general population, people with T1DM have more than twice the risk of fracture. Episodes of hypoglycemia increase fracture risk by more than 50%. Insulin treatment does not change the risk of fracture [25].

Hypoglycemia has a profound negative effect on the quality of life for individuals with diabetes. Patients who experience frequent episodes of symptomatic hypoglycemia within a year reported making significant lifestyle adjustments. These adjustments include avoiding social settings and structuring daily activities around meal and medication schedules [26]. Consequently, individuals with a history of severe hypoglycemia demonstrate lower scores on assessments of overall health and well-being, including the EQ-5D Visual Analog Scale, World Health Organization Five Well-Being Index, Problem Areas in Diabetes Scale, and Food Habits Questionnaire. Additionally, the fear of hypoglycemia becomes a self-perpetuating concern. Experiencing one or more severe hypoglycemic episodes within a year doubles the likelihood of scoring within the highest tertile of the Fear of Hypoglycemia Questionnaire [27].

2.2 Pathophysiology of hypoglycemia

2.2.1 Risk factors for hypoglycemia

Hypoglycemia may arise from an excess of therapeutic insulin or a failure in defense mechanisms against a decrease in plasma glucose concentration. Common risk factors for iatrogenic hypoglycemia (**Table 1**) include missed or insufficient meals in relation to insulin therapy, unaccustomed physical exertion without additional caloric intake, overall improvements in fitness and insulin sensitivity without adjusting the insulin dosage, and other instances of inadvertent or misguided insulin overdosage. Other contributing factors comprise alcohol consumption, which inhibits gluconeogenesis; drug interactions; systemic illnesses linked to malnutrition or poor food intake; chronic liver disease (resulting in impaired glucose production); and renal failure (accompanied by decreases in renal gluconeogenesis and insulin clearance).

In individuals without diabetes, a decrease in plasma glucose prompts a swift reduction in insulin secretion. This diminished insulin secretion limits peripheral glucose disposal, initiates lipolysis (thus providing gluconeogenic substrates), and enables two essential hepatic processes: glycogenolysis and gluconeogenesis. The reduction in insulin secretion is a crucial physiological response designed to elevate plasma glucose back to the normal range. However, individuals with T1DM, lacking the capacity for autoregulation of insulin secretion, experience unavoidable fluctuations in exogenous insulin administration and caloric intake. Those with insulin deficiency (C-peptide negative) lack endogenous insulin that can be suppressed in reaction to declining plasma glucose levels. Paradoxically, the insulin deficiency that underlies hyperglycemia in T1DM patients becomes a primary risk factor for iatrogenic hypoglycemia [28].

In individuals with T1DM who are incapable of suppressing circulating (exogenous) insulin levels, pharmacokinetic factors serve as the sole mechanism for eliminating administered insulin during evolving hypoglycemia. To put it succinctly, there are presently no strategies to directly hinder the action or expedite the removal of injected insulin. Furthermore, conditions that impair insulin clearance (such as renal failure) increase the risk of prolonged hypoglycemia.

2.2.2 Other risk factors for hypoglycemia

Additional risk factors for hypoglycemia in individuals with T1DM encompass a history of severe hypoglycemia, the pursuit of intensive glycemic control, hypoglycemia unawareness, and low levels of HbA1C. Deficiencies in glucocorticoids, such as those seen in Addison's disease, heighten insulin sensitivity, escalating the risk of severe or recurrent insulin-induced hypoglycemia. Furthermore, polymorphisms

Inadequate caloric consumption	Increased insulin sensitivity	Impaired glucose production
Skipped meals	Weight loss	Alcohol intake
Delayed meals	Exercise	Liver disease
Malnutrition	Improved fitness	Renal failure
Intercurrent illness	Medications	

Table 1.
Common risk factors for hypoglycemia in T1DM [28].

in the angiotensin-converting enzyme (ACE) gene have been proposed as potential contributors to the risk of severe hypoglycemia in individuals with T1DM [29]. Genotypes at two variants of ADRB2 (Adrenoceptor Beta 2) are associated with impaired awareness of hypoglycemia [30].

2.2.3 Impairment in counter-regulatory responses to hypoglycemia

A reduction in plasma glucose concentration typically elicits two primary responses in the body under normal circumstances: [1] Elevated endogenous glucose production through processes such as glycogenolysis and gluconeogenesis and [2] Behavioral changes, including sensations of hunger and a tendency to seek food.

In individuals without diabetes, the initial response to a decline in glucose concentration involves a reduction in insulin secretion, occurring while the glucose concentration is still within the lower physiological range. As the glucose concentration approaches or falls just below the physiological range, other counter-regulatory hormones are released. Glucagon, discharged by pancreatic alpha cells into the hepatic portal circulation, experiences an approximate increase within 15 minutes once the glycemic threshold is reached. Its hyperglycemic effects are realized through the stimulation of glycogenolysis, gluconeogenesis, and lipolysis, resulting in an augmentation of hepatic glucose production. Glucagon is released at a glucose threshold of around 68 mg/dl (3.7 mmol/L) and plays a pivotal role in promptly rectifying hypoglycemia. It is indispensable for achieving complete restoration of normoglycemia subsequent to insulin administration.

When plasma glucose levels reach approximately 69–70 mg/dl (3.8 mmol/L), the release of epinephrine can occur, typically increasing around 20 minutes after reaching this threshold. Epinephrine exerts its effects by stimulating hepatic glycogenolysis and gluconeogenesis, enhancing glycolysis in muscles, and promoting lipolysis in adipose tissue. Additionally, it restricts glucose utilization by reducing insulin secretion and diminishing glucose uptake.

The function of secondary counterregulatory hormones, such as cortisol and growth hormone, is relatively modest and not crucial. Interestingly, hypercortisolemia appears to weaken symptomatic, autonomic, and neuroendocrine responses to subsequent hypoglycemia. Due to the underlying destruction of pancreatic β-cells in patients with T1DM, autoregulation of insulin secretion is not feasible during decreasing plasma glucose levels. However, the other counterregulatory responses occur to varying extents. Counterregulatory responses, especially sympathetic activation, are accountable for the autonomic warning symptoms of impending hypoglycemia. In this context, counter-regulation and awareness are physiologically intertwined in the earliest stages of defense against emerging hypoglycemia. Patients with impaired glucose counter-regulation may experience a decrease in counterregulatory hormone secretion during hypoglycemia, resulting in the absence of typical warning symptoms that accompany milder degrees of hypoglycemia.

The mentioned defense mechanisms are often compromised in patients with diabetes, and significant beta-cell failure is associated with the absence of an initial response to a decline in insulin. This leads to a delay in glucose secretion from the liver during hypoglycemia. The frequency of hypoglycemic episodes increases with the duration of diabetes, possibly due to the gradual decline in endogenous insulin. This decline occurs more rapidly in patients with T1DM and at a slower pace in those with T2DM. Additionally, although it is normal in the initial stages of diabetes, the glucagon reaction to hypoglycemia deteriorates over time in T1DM and more slowly in

T2DM. For unclear reasons, glucagon-releasing responses to hypoglycemia disappear within approximately 5 years of T1DM diagnosis, leaving epinephrine responses as the only early defense against hypoglycemia. Interestingly, epinephrine responses to hypoglycemia are attenuated by ~50% in patients with T1DM compared with healthy subjects. Epinephrine and other counterregulatory responses can be blunted by a single episode of hypoglycemia, worsened by recurrent episodes of hypoglycemia, and reversed by rigorous avoidance of iatrogenic hypoglycemia.

Essentially, iatrogenic hypoglycemia is the outcome of the interaction between insulin excess and impaired glucose counter-regulation in patients with T1DM.

2.2.4 Hypoglycemia unawareness

Hypoglycemia unawareness in diabetes is characterized by the inability to recognize the symptoms of impending hypoglycemia by a patient. This condition is particularly associated with effective glycemic control.

Recurrent hypoglycemia may arise due to a diminished autonomic response to hypoglycemia, leading to a reduction in autonomic warning symptoms. The impaired brain response is marked by increased GLUT1 activity, aiming to preserve brain function and modifying glucose sensing in the ventromedial hypothalamus through elevated levels of gamma-aminobutyric acid.

Partial or complete hypoglycemia unawareness is observed in 25–50% of patients with T1DM and is strongly correlated with a prolonged duration of diabetes, typically exceeding 20 years. This state has been defined by Cryer as hypoglycemia-associated autonomic failure (HAAF) [31].

HAAF and impaired awareness of hypoglycemia (IAH) are clinical concepts that describe frequent and recent exposure to iatrogenic hypoglycemia in patients with T1DM. This exposure leads to a defective counter-regulatory hormonal response, especially the epinephrine response, as well as hypoglycemia unawareness. Intensive glycemic therapy with tight glycemic control has been associated with an increased risk of developing HAAF [32]. Moreover, individuals with HAAF face a sixfold elevated risk of iatrogenic hypoglycemia [33]. Additionally, both exercise and sleep can enhance the diminished autonomic response [34].

Multiple theories have been postulated, including: [1] the systemic–mediator hypothesis, suggesting that elevated circulating cortisol during hypoglycemia diminishes the sympathoadrenal and symptomatic response to subsequent hypoglycemia; [2] the brain fuel–transport hypothesis, proposing that recent hypoglycemia leads to increased blood-to-brain transport of glucose or alternative fuels, thereby attenuating sympathoadrenal and symptomatic responses to subsequent hypoglycemia; [3] the brain–metabolism hypothesis, stating that recent hypoglycemia alters CNS metabolic regulation, resulting in subdued sympathoadrenal responses; and [4] the cerebral network hypothesis, which posits that recent hypoglycemia acts through a network of interconnected brain regions mediated through the thalamus to inhibit hypothalamic activation, thus attenuating the sympatho-adrenal and symptomatic responses to subsequent hypoglycemia [35]. Hence, a complex interplay exists between central and peripheral mechanisms to sense and respond appropriately to declining blood glucose levels. **Figure 1** shows the mechanisms associated with HAAF in patients with T1DM.

The hyperinsulinemic hypoglycemic clamp technique is considered the gold standard for evaluating impaired awareness of hypoglycemia (IAH). This method involves measuring hypoglycemic symptoms at specified intervals during the clamp procedure as plasma glucose levels are systematically lowered. Individuals who do not

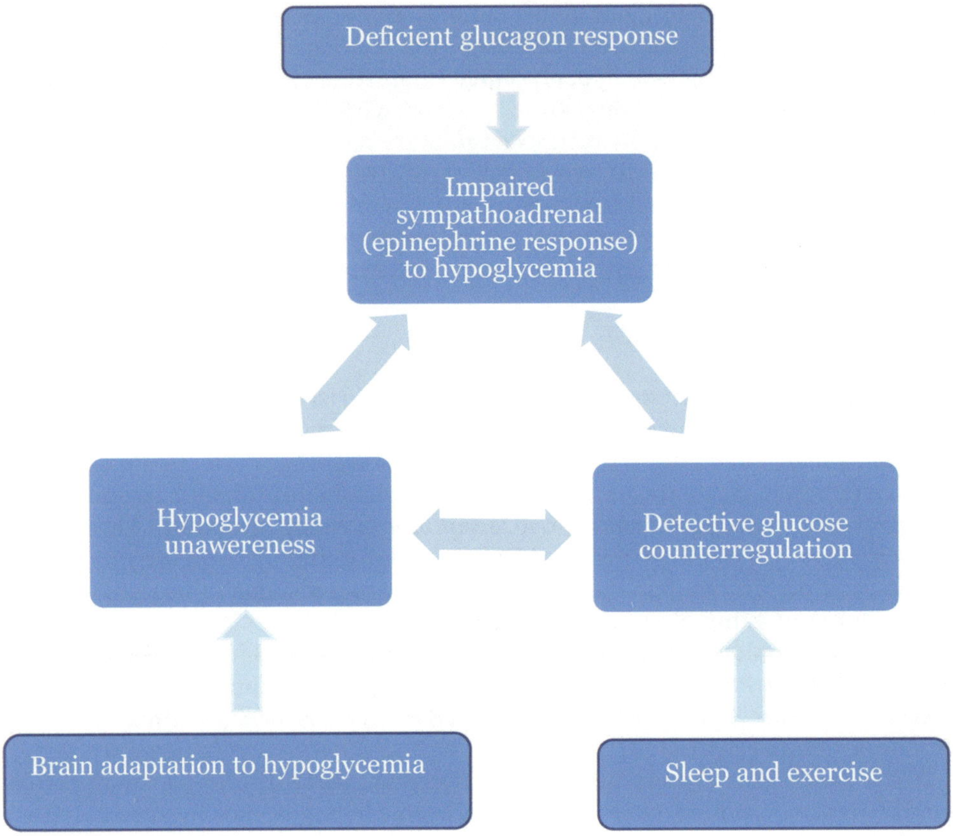

Figure 1.
Mechanisms associated with HAAF in patients with T1DM.

exhibit significant hypoglycemic symptoms, even around glucose levels of 50–54 mg/dl, are classified as having IAH. While this technique is an objective and well-established approach for assessing hypoglycemia and counter-regulation mechanisms, its application is primarily confined to research studies.

Numerous questionnaires have been formulated and extensively employed, primarily for research endeavors, to evaluate IAH. These include the Gold, Clarke, Pedersen-Bjergaard, Hypo or Ryan, DAFNE IAH, and HypoA-Q scores [36]. Self-reported hypoglycemia awareness questionnaires are relatively inexpensive and easy to administer. However, they are susceptible to recall and reporting biases, and their incorporation into research studies or clinical care has not been standardized. Combining clinical questionnaires with continuous glucose monitoring (CGM) data in diabetes mellitus management has demonstrated an improved specificity for identifying individuals with longstanding T1DM and a lack of autonomic symptom recognition in response to insulin-induced hypoglycemia [36, 37].

2.3 Clinical manifestations of hypoglycemia

The clinical manifestations of hypoglycemia include asymptomatic, mild, and severe episodes. Asymptomatic episodes of hypoglycemia manifest in patients with IAH and are most effectively diagnosed through self-blood glucose monitoring

(SMBG) data. Unreported incidents of mild and severe hypoglycemia commonly occur during sleep in individuals with T1DM [28]. Nocturnal hypoglycemia is prevalent due to the fact that individuals in a sleep state are typically in a post-absorptive or fasting condition and are often deprived of calories [28].

Mild episodes of hypoglycemia respond promptly to appropriate measures and seem not to leave clinically detectable sequelae. However, even milder degrees of hypoglycemia have been reported to induce measurable impairments in brain stem function. Severe hypoglycemia has the potential to induce seizures, physical harm, or coma. Depending on the context (e.g., in traffic or while operating machinery), secondary damage may also occur. Recurrent, severe, or prolonged hypoglycemia can lead to permanent cognitive impairment or death. To mitigate the risk of nocturnal hypoglycemia, it is advisable for individuals undergoing intensive therapy to incorporate occasional nocturnal time points (between 2 and 5 am) into their SMBG protocol. Other predictable periods characterized by an elevated frequency of iatrogenic hypoglycemia include interprandial intervals and the post-exercise period [28].

2.3.1 Symptoms of hypoglycemia

Symptoms of hypoglycemia encompass autonomic symptoms and neuroglycopenic symptoms, exhibiting variation among patients based on age and diabetes duration. In the case of children, emotional and behavioral changes may manifest alongside classic autonomic and neuroglycopenic symptoms. Autonomic symptoms entail sweating, palpitations, tremulousness, hunger, and nervousness, while neuroglycopenic symptoms comprise impaired concentration, tiredness, dizziness/faintness, confusion, convulsions, seizures, tingling, and blurred vision [28]. Neuroglycopenic symptoms arise from the deprivation of glucose to brain neurons. The glycemic threshold for the onset of neuroglycopenic symptoms is typically around 54 mg/dL. [11, 38].

3. The management of hypoglycemia in type 1 diabetes mellitus

Previous experience of hypoglycemia and fear of hypoglycemia are the key barriers that prevent patients with T1DM from using their medical treatment properly in the optimization of glycemic control. For minimizing the risk of hypoglycemia, patient education, reducing the conventional risk factors for hypoglycemia, and minimizing the risk factors indicative of HAAF are the main steps.

3.1 Patient education

The anticipation, recognition, and treatment of hypoglycemia by patients with T1DM is fundamentally important. They should recognize their most commonly encountered symptoms of hypoglycemia, learn how to manage hypoglycemia and learn the predisposing risk factors for hypoglycemia. The patient should be educated about SMBG (including nocturnal testing) and counting carbohydrates to permit a flexible diet. There are many studies in the literature evaluating the effect of patient education on hypoglycemia [39–42]. In some studies, participation in the diabetes teaching and treatment program (DTTP) improved HbA1C while reducing severe hypoglycemia by approximately 50% [39–41]. Hopkins et al. reported improved awareness of hypoglycemia in up to 43% of participants at

1 year follow-up with DTTP [41], and the rate of IAH decreased from 39.9–33%, with improvement in psychological distress and well-being up to 1 year following DTTP [41]. In the HypoCOMPaSS trial, a half-day education about reducing episodes of hypoglycemia was given to all participants [42]. At 6 months, all groups reached great improvement in IAH, and rates of severe hypoglycemia fell from 77–20% at the end of the 6-month trial (8.9 ± 13.4 vs. 0.8 ± 1.8 episodes per person per year; $p = 0.0001$) [42]. All these studies show that structured education (defined as insulin self-management and/or specific training for the avoidance of hypoglycemia) is effective in decreasing the rates of severe hypoglycemia in T1DM with improvement in glycemic control. In every documented hypoglycemia, the conditions of the event should be evaluated together with the patient to try to find out the etiology of hypoglycemia, for example, a skipped meal/prolonged fasting, physical exertion, alcohol consumption, and injection of a high insulin dose. Patient support should be provided by a team including professionals trained in glycemic management, and caregivers should work with each individual patient over time to find the best methods to prevent hypoglycemia.

3.2 Dietary intervention

Dietary intervention includes information about the amount of carbohydrates at meals and their influence on blood glucose levels and forming an individualized regular meal plan. The patients using insulin should be educated about the appropriate dosage and time of insulin in relation to meals. Patients at risk of hypoglycemia should be notified always to keep glucose or foods containing carbohydrates at hand.

3.3 Frequent SMBG

Patients should be educated about how to apply SMBG in their daily practice. Patients with T1DM should perform SMBG regularly and whenever they suspect hypoglycemia. Especially before performing a critical task such as driving, it is crucial to check their glucose level. SMBG documents hypo/hyperglycemia and allows patients to correlate their symptoms and glucose levels. Moreover, patients adjust their regimen according to the provided data from SMBG to prevent hypoglycemia. Paired glucose testing before and 2 hours after meals should be measured during SMBG. Normally, the difference between the premeal and 2-hour postprandial glucose should be <50 mg/dL. If the difference between these values is negative at 2 hours, the patient is likely to become hypoglycemic by 3 hours after eating, so the patient should be advised to check their blood glucose level again.

3.4 Individualized glycemic goals

To achieve a target a HbA1C level of 6.5%, fasting plasma glucose (FPG) should be kept at <110 mg/dL and 2-hour postprandial glucose (PPG) <140 mg/dL [43]. It is not always possible to achieve that level without hypoglycemia. If a patient has limited life expectancy, a history of severe hypoglycemia and/or hypoglycemia unawareness, advanced renal disease or other severe comorbid conditions with a high risk for CVD events and prohibitive cognitive and/or psychological status, it is not necessary to control strictly blood glucose levels. Instead, a less stringent A1C target (e.g., 7–8%) becomes reasonable [43].

3.5 Newer insulins

The use of a long-acting basal insulin analog (glargine, detemir) rather than NPH insulin in an MDI regimen is reported to reduce hypoglycemia including nocturnal hypoglycemia in patients with T1DM [44, 45]. Rapid-acting analogs (lispro, aspart, and glulisine) with faster onset and shortened duration of action are found to be associated with a 20% reduction in the risk of severe hypoglycemia and nocturnal hypoglycemia compared to regular insulin in patients with T1DM [44, 45]. A randomized trial including patients with IAH demonstrated a 29% reduction in the number of episodes of severe hypoglycemia per person-year with an insulin analog-based regimen when compared to a regimen of regular insulin and NPH [46]. Recently introduced ultra-fast-acting analogs may reduce this risk further [47]. They have faster onset of action and shorter exposure times. The PRONTO-T1D study compared the ultra-rapid lispro (URLi) with lispro in 269 patients with T1DM and found that both mealtime URLi and URLi given after the meal were associated with significant reductions in nocturnal hypoglycemia and decreased time spent in hypoglycemia compared with mealtime lispro [48]. Moreover, longer-acting basal insulins with less day-to-day variability (insulin degludec four times↓ day-to-day variability vs. U-100 glargine) and reduced nocturnal peak action (insulin degludec and U-300 glargine) have been associated with a reduced risk of nocturnal and severe hypoglycemia [49, 50].

3.6 Minimizing the conventional risk factors for hypoglycemia

Ill-timed insulin is a major problem in the glycemic control management. Patients should be educated about the proper timing of insulin dosing in relation to meals. Insulin analogs should be injected 5–15 minutes prior to meal time. If the preprandial glucose is <80 mg/dL, the injection should be done at the beginning of the meal. Patients with T1DM should be aware of "insulin stacking," a condition whereby patients inject bolus insulin prior to complete absorption of prior insulin dose. The general rule for insulin analogs is that 90, 60, and 40% of the insulin remain on board after 1, 2, and 3 hours following a bolus of the insulin, respectively.

3.7 Reducing the risk factors indicative of HAAF

Patients with HAAF should have higher targeted fasting and postprandial glucose values as well as HbA1C levels >7%. With a history of HA, a 2- to 3-week trial of scrupulous avoidance of hypoglycemia is advised to restore awareness. These patients should also be initiated on glucose sensors, notifying them with an alarm system.

3.8 Insulin pump therapy

Continuous subcutaneous insulin infusion (CSII) via an insulin pump allows insulin delivery, supplying variable doses according to the time of the day. Insulin pumps comprise four parts: [1] the infusion site, [2] the reservoir, [3] the pump, and [4] the control and interface (with sensor-augmented pump and hybrid closed-loop pumps). There is controversial data about the benefit of CSII in the prevention of hypoglycemia in the literature. In a meta-analysis including 19 studies comparing MDI with CSII, comparable rates of severe hypoglycemia between the groups were reported [51]. On the other hand, another meta-analysis demonstrated a 4.2-fold reduction in SH incidence in CSII users rather than MDI users [52]. The Relative Effectiveness of Pumps Over MDI and Structured Education (REPOSE) trial, which is the largest and the longest randomized controlled trial (RCT) of CSII in T1DM, compared the patients receiving insulin by either CSII or MDI after structured education [53]. In both groups, improvement in HbA1C and severe hypoglycemia (50%↓) was achieved, and structured education is advocated in flexible insulin self-management before progression to CSII for hypoglycemia [53].

3.9 CGM

Continuous glucose monitoring (CGM) has provided a major advance in the treatment of persons with all forms of DM to reach goals safely. The first CGM system was released by Medtronic in 1999 [CGMS Gold, Medtronic, Inc., North-ridge, CA [54]]. These systems measure the glucose levels in interstitial fluid space in 1- or 5-minute increments with a lag of 4–10 min. The device has three components: a disposable sensor measuring the current glucose, a transmitter attached to the sensor, and a receiver displaying and storing glucose information. A sensor wire (size: 21G to 26G) is inserted under the skin using an applicator or insertion device. The transmitter sends a radio frequency signal to the receiver, where it is translated into a glucose value. The accuracy of the sensor is checked by periodic calibration using capillary blood glucose obtained from a fingerstick in 3-, 5-, or 7-day intervals, depending on the system.

CGM can be categorized into two classes: blinded retrospective CGM and real-time CGM. In blinded type CGM, glucose measurement is done intermittently to collect data on glucose excursion and facilitate changes in therapy, while real-time CGM displays current glucose value with alerts and alarms to intervene and manage their diabetes in response to impending hypo/hyperglycemia. In many countries, CGM is approved for use in all persons with DM on multiple-dose insulin (3 injections/day) or an insulin pump as well as those who have frequent or severe hypoglycemia, nocturnal hypoglycemia, or hypoglycemia unawareness. At present, three types of CGM systems are available: retrospective CGM (r-CGM), real-time glucose monitoring (rt-CGM), and intermittent scanning CGM (isCGM). Rt-CGM devices in which readers, either stand-alone devices or integrated into insulin pumps or mobile phones, show transmitted interstitial glucose readings in real-time, whereas isCGM devices demonstrate glucose values on demand when the sensor is scanned with a reading device. Rt-CGM or isCGM including alarms or alerts is recommended particularly for persons with hypoglycemia who would benefit from these warnings. **Table 2** summarizes the main characteristics of currently available CGM sensor devices.

CGM can be used independently to guide therapy or integrated with an insulin pump called sensor-augmented pump (SAP) therapy. SAP therapy with a glucose suspend (LGS) property automatically stops insulin delivery in response to hypoglycemia for up to 2 hr. and restarts it upon recovery (e.g., MiniMed 640G SAP system, Medtronic. Inc.). The Food and Drug Administration approved using the first closed-loop system, the MiniMed 670G System (Medtronic), for patients 14 years or older in the United States in 2016.

A hybrid closed-loop system (HCL) is like an artificial pancreas. It manages an insulin delivery automatically without patient intervention. The system calculates insulin dosages continually related to CGM levels by using a proprietary proportional-integral-derivative controller. Many studies evaluating the effect of closed-loop systems on glycemic control have shown that the rate of hypoglycemia and severe hypoglycemia is decreased in both adults and children, especially at nighttime [55, 56].

CGM system	Manufacturer	Accuracy (MARD)%	Calibrations	Sensor lifetime, day	Smart features	Limitations
Enlite-Sensor	Medtronic	13.6	Every 12 hr	6	Trend arrows, rate-of-change alerts, hypo/hyperglycemic alarms	Acetaminophen interference
Guardian Sensor 3	Medtronic	10.6 (abdomen) 9.1 (arm)	Every 12 hr	7	Trend arrows, rate-of-change alerts, hypo/hyperglycemic alarms	Acetaminophen interference
Freestyle Navigator II	Abbott	14.5	2, 10, 24, 72 hr. after insertion	5	Trend arrows, rate-of-change alerts, hypo/hyperglycemic alarms	
Freestyle Libre	Abbott	11.4	No	14	Trend arrows	Sensor need to be scanned to get a glucose reading, not recommended for patients with IHA
Freestyle Libre 2	Abbott	NA	No	14	Trend arrows, rate-of-change alerts, hypo/hyperglycemic alarms, remote monitoring	Sensor need to be scanned to get a glucose reading, not recommended for patients with IHA
G4 Platinum	Dexcom	9	Every 12 hr	7	Trend arrows, rate-of-change alerts, hypo/hyperglycemic alarms, remote monitoring	
G5 Mobile	Dexcom	9	Every 12 hr	7	Trend arrows, rate-of-change alerts, hypo/hyperglycemic alarms, remote monitoring, wireless communication up to five devices	Acetaminophen interference
G6	Dexcom	10	Every 12 hr	10	Trend arrows, rate-of-change alerts, hypo/hyperglycemic alarms, remote monitoring, wireless communication up to five devices	
Eversense	Senseonics	11.4	No	90	Trend arrows, rate-of-change alerts, hypo/hyperglycemic alarms	The sensor should be inserted and removed in doctor's office

Table 2.
Summary of the main characteristics of the CGM sensor devices.

In an open-label, randomized, crossover study, the use of a closed-loop system significantly increased the time in range (TIR), whereas the time spent in hypoglycemic range significantly decreased during both daytime and nighttime in adolescents with T1DM [56]. It is one of the most promising technologies to attain optimal glycemic control, minimizing the episodes of hypoglycemia and severe hypoglycemia, particularly at nighttime. Although the majority of the systems include single-hormone insulin, dual-hormone systems, which infuse both insulin and glucagon, have also been in the research phase [57, 58].

There are many randomized controlled trials (RCTs) evaluating the potential benefit of CGM in the management of T1DM and the prevention of problematic hypoglycemia. **Table 3** shows the summary of these RCTs.

These studies showed that continuous use and high compliance are very necessary to achieve maximum glucose-lowering effect with CGM. Moreover, the DIAMOND and GOLD studies show that CGM is also beneficial for patients on conventional MDI treatment [61, 62]. A recent meta-analysis evaluating the effectiveness of GCM in the regulation of diabetes mellitus included 21 studies involving 2149 individuals [77]. In this meta-analysis, it is found that CGM significantly decreased HbA1C levels compared with SMBG (mean difference −2.46 mmol/mol, p: 0.0005) and is especially effective in Type 1 diabetic patients with uncontrolled glycemia (HbA1C > 8%) [77]. On the other hand, CGM was reported to have no influence on the number of severe hypoglycemia cases (p: 0.13) in this meta-analysis [77]. Maiorino et al. reported a meta-analysis of 15 RCTs, including 2461 patients, comparing CGM with usual care in both type 1 and type 2 diabetes mellitus on the effect of glycemic control [78]. In this study, it is shown that CGM was associated with a modest reduction in HbA1C (−0.17%, 95% CI -0.29 to −0.06, I^2: 96.2%), increase in TIR (70.74 min, 95% CI 46.73–94.76, I^2: 66.3%), and lower time above range (TIR) and time below range (TBR) with heterogeneity between studies [78]. In subgroup analyses, rt-CGM led to a higher improvement in mean HbA1C (−0.23%, 95% CI -0.36 to −0.10, p < 0.001), TIR (83.49 min, 95% CI 52.68–114.30, P < 0.001), and TAR, whereas both is-CGM and SAP were associated with the greater decline in TBR [78]. In another meta-analysis by Wang et al., 10 RCTs and 5 crossover design trials, with a total of 2071 patients were included [79]. In this meta-analysis, it is demonstrated that CGM is effective in reducing HbA1C levels (−2.69%, 95% CI (−4.25 to −1.14), p < 0.001) and decreasing the incidence of SH events (RR: 0.52, 95% CI 0.35–0.77; p: 0:001) [79].

The impact of CGM on quality of life is studied in many studies in the literature. The GOLD study reported a significant improvement in QoL in CGM-treated patients when compared to controls [61]. In this study, a significant improvement in patient well-being assessed using the WHO-5 questionnaire (66.1 vs. 62.7, p: 0.02) and in treatment satisfaction assessed using the Diabetes Treatment Satisfaction Questionnaire (DTSQ) (30.21 vs. 26.62, P < 0.001) with less hypoglycemia fear assessed using the Hypoglycemia Confidence Questionnaire (HCQ) scale (3.40 vs. 3.27, p < 0.001) was shown with CGM use [61]. Klak et al. compared the emotional well-being of adults with T1DM between CGM users and SMBG users in a meta-analysis including 11 studies involving 1228 patients with T1DM [80]. This meta-analysis showed that CGM systems reduced fear of hypoglycemia (Cohen d = −0.24; 95% CI, −0.41 to −0.07; p: 0.005) and increased patient satisfaction with improved quality of life [80].

In many studies, it has been emphasized that >80% compliance is needed to reach optimum benefit with CGM [61–63, 81]. However, compliance is a great problem while using CGM. A major problem is discomfort while wearing the CGM (42%),

DOI: http://dx.doi.org/10.5772/intechopen.1004108

Study	Intervention	Participants (N)	Impact on hypoglycemia	HbA1C change	Duration of follow-up	Adherence to CGM (%)
JDRF study [59]	CGM vs. SMBG	322 participants Children 8–14 yrs. Young adults 15–24 yrs. Adults>25 yrs	No difference in SH events	0.5%↓-Adults No change in the young group	26 weeks	The young group-50%↓
Battelino et al. [60]	CGM vs. SMBG	120 patients (HbA1C <7.5%)	↓Time spent in hypoglycemia (0.48–0.57 vs. 0.97–1.55 h/day) ($p = 0.03$)	0.21%↓ (p: 0.008)	26 weeks	
GOLD study [61]	CGM vs. SMBG (Dexcom G4 Platinum)	161 patients (HbA1C ≥7.5% on MDI)	↓Hypoglycemia (2.79 vs. 4.79%). ↓ SH events (5 vs. 1)	7.92% (7.79 to 8.05) vs. 8.35% (8.19 to 8.51) ($p < 0.001$)	26 weeks	87.8%
DIAMOND study [62]	CGM vs. SMBG (Dexcom G4 Platinum)	158 patients (HbA1C 7.5–9.9% on MDI)	↓Time spent in hypoglycemia (43 min/day vs. 80 min/day) ($p = 0.002$) No difference in SH events (2 vs. 2)	1.1% vs.0.5↓- 12 wks 1.0% vs. 0.4↓- 24 wks ($p < 0.01$)	24 weeks	93%
IMPACT study [63]	FGM vs. SMBG	328 patients (HbA1C ≤ 7.5%)	38% ↓ in time in hypoglycemia	No difference in HbA1C	6 months	
JDRF<7 study [64]	CGM vs. SMBG	129 adults and children (age range 8–69 years) HbA1C < 7.0%	Median time with a glucose level ≤ 60 mg/dl (18 vs. 35 min/day, $p = 0.05$) Time out of range (377 vs. 491 min/day, $p = 0.003$) No difference in SH events ($p = 1.0$)	6.4 ± 0.5 vs.6.8 ± 0.5 ($p < 0.001$)	26 weeks	67%↓ in final 4 weeks
IN CONTROL study [65]	CGM vs. SMBG	52 patients with IAH (Gold score > 4)	↓Time spent in hypoglycemia (6.8% vs. 11.4%) ↓SH events (14 vs. 34 events, $P = 0.033$)	−0·1% vs. -0.1% (p: 0.449)	16 wks -CGM 12 wks -wash-out	

Study	Intervention	Participants (N)	Impact on hypoglycemia	HbA1C change	Duration of follow-up	Adherence to CGM (%)
The Real Trend study [66]	rt-CGM (SAP) vs. SMBG	132 adults and children (HbA1C ≥8%)	No difference in hypoglycemia	In fully compliant patients CGM group -↓0.96%– 0.93% CSII group - ↓0.55%– 0.93%, (P < 0.004)	6 months	>25 yrs. 74.9% 5–14 yrs. 68.4% 15–25 yrs. 52.4%
SMILE study [67]	rt-CGM (SAP) vs. SMBG	153 patients (HbA1C 5·8–10·0% and Gold score > 4)	↓Hypoglycemic events per week (−2·9 [95% CI -3·5 to −2·3]) (p < 0·0001) ↓SH events (3 vs. 18; p = 0·0036)	No difference in HbA1C	24 wks	
HypoDE study [68]	rt-CGM (SAP) vs. SMBG	148 patients with IAH	↓Hypoglycemic events (10·8 to 3·5 /28 days) 72%↓ in hypoglycemic events	No difference in HbA1C	26 wks	
Jensen et al. [69]	P-CGM vs. SMBG	472 patients	↓Symptomatic hypoglycemia (0.82; 95% CI: 0.69–0.97) ↓Asymptomatic hypoglycemia (0.72; 95% CI: 0.53–0.97) ↓Time spent in hypoglycemia (p: 0.0070)	Less glycemic variability (p: 0.0043) No difference in HbA1C (0.06%, p: 0.2028)	16 wks	
Laffel et al. [70]	rt-CGM vs. SMBG	153 patients (age range 14-24 years) (HbA1C 7.5%–10.9%)	↓Mean time in hypoglycemia −0.7% [95% CI, −1.5% to −0.1%] (p: 0.002) No difference in SH (3 vs. 2)	Adjusted between-group difference −0.37% [95% CI, −0.66% to −0.08%] (p: 0.01)	26 wks	

DOI: http://dx.doi.org/10.5772/intechopen.1004108

Study	Intervention	Participants (N)	Impact on hypoglycemia	HbA1C change	Duration of follow-up	Adherence to CGM (%)
Pratley et al. [71]	rt-CGM vs. SMBG	203 patients	↓Mean time in hypoglycemia −1.9% (−27 minutes per day) ($p < 0.001$)	Adjusted group difference, −0.3%; (95% CI, −0.4% to −0.1%) $p < 0.001$	24 wks	
Zhang et al. [72]	FGM vs. SMBG	146 patients	↓The duration of hypoglycemia (p < 0.05) ↑TIR [(49.39 ± 17.54)% vs. (42.44 ± 15.49)%] (p: 0.012)	8.16 ± 1.03 vs. 8.68 ± 1.01 (p: 0.003)	48 wks	
HypoCOMPaSS study [42]	rt-CGM vs. SMBG	96 patients	↓The duration of hypoglycemia (53 ± 63 to 24 ± 56 min/24 h (*p*: 0.004) ↑Hypoglycemia awareness (5.1 ± 1.1 to 4.1 ± 1.6; *p*: 0.0001) ↓SH (8.9 ± 13.4 to 0.8 ± 1.8 episodes/patient-year) (*p*: 0.0001)	↓0.3%-No difference in HbA1C	24 wks	
STAR3 study [73]	rt-CGM (SAP) vs. SMBG	485 patients (329 adults and 156 children)	No change in the rate of SH	↓ HbA1C (7.4% vs. 8.0%, P < 0.001)	24 wks	
SWITCH study [74]	CGM (SAP) vs. SMBG	153 patients (adults and children) (HbA1C 7.5% - 9.5%)	↓time spent in hypoglycemia (19 vs. 31 min/day; p = 0.009) No difference in SH events (4 vs. 2; p = 0·4)	↓-0.43% in HbA1C (8.04% vs. 8.47%) (p < 0.001)	24 wks	

Study	Intervention	Participants (N)	Impact on hypoglycemia	HbA1C change	Duration of follow-up	Adherence to CGM (%)
ASPIRE study [75]	rt-CGM (SAP with LGS) vs. SMBG	247 patients	↓37.5% in mean AUC for nocturnal hypoglycemic events ↓ 31.8% nocturnal hypoglycemic events	No difference in HbA1C	3 months	
Ly et al. [76]	rt-CGM (SAP with LGS) vs. SMBG	95 patients Mean age 18.6 yrs	↓ Hypoglycemic events (175 to 35 vs. 28 to 16)	No difference in HbA1C	24 wks	
APCam11 study Jasleen [56]	HCL vs. SAP	86 patients (11–36 yrs)	↓time spent in hypoglycemia (p:0.013)	↓ 0.36% in HbA1C ($p < 0.001$)	12 wks	
iDCL study Jasleen [55]	CL (SAP with LGS) vs. SAP	168 patients (14–71 yrs)	time spent in hypoglycemia ($p < 0.001$)	↓ 0.33% in HbA1C ($p < 0.001$)	26 wks	

Table 3.
RCTs about the benefits of CGM in the management of hypoglycemia in T1DM.

followed by problems with CGM insertion (33%), problems with adhesion to skin (30%), poor performance (28%), alarms (27%), accuracy (25%) interference with sports and activities (18%), and skin reactions from the CGM sensor (18%). Flash glucose monitoring (FGM) is associated with less discomfort and side effects (less pain, less bleeding on sensor insertion, less itching, and less erythema). Some of the features of FGM differ from the existing sensor technology. FGM measures interstitial glucose levels for up to 14 days without calibration by fingerstick blood glucose measurements, and the wireless handheld reader scans the sensor every 15 minutes for up to 8 hr. to receive the glucose values. Along with factory calibration and no alarm system, FGM may be an attractive option with higher rates of compliance.

The accuracy of the CGM is a great concern for CGM users. It is measured using the mean absolute relative differences (MARDs) between CGM readings and blood glucose readings. The physiological lag time between interstitial and blood glucose, which is usually between 4 and 10 min, can be longer when glucose concentrations are changing rapidly. Also, when the decrease in glucose levels is rapid on approaching hypoglycemic levels, the sensor can show falsely higher values. While early CGM devices had a high error rate with MARDs of around 20%, these error rates are now between 9 and 14% with advances in sensor technology. The MARD of the flash glucose monitoring system (FGS) system is 11.4%, whereas the latest Dexcom G5 system is just under 10%.

3.10 Islet cell transplantation

For patients with resistant hypoglycemia despite all the therapies mentioned above, islet cell transplantation may be an option. In a phase 3 study by the Clinical Islet Transplantation Consortium in North America, including 48 adults with T1DM and IAH, improvement in glycemic control and a significant decrease in SH events (2 events, $p < 0.0003$) was achieved after islet cell transplantation [82].

4. Treatment of hypoglycemia in type 1 DM

4.1 Oral self-treatment

In case of hypoglycemia, glucose tablets, juice, soft drinks, or candy, containing 15–20 g glucose should be taken by the patient with T1DM. After 15–20 minutes, blood glucose should be checked, and if it is still <80 mg/dl, 15–20 g glucose should be repeated until the blood glucose level is over>80 mg/dl. Since the glycemic response is transient, the patient should be given a subsequent more substantial snack or meal.

4.2 Parenteral treatment

When a hypoglycemic patient is unable to take carbohydrates orally because of loss of consciousness, parenteral therapy is needed. Glucagon is usually injected subcutaneously or intramuscularly by a partner of the patient who has learned to treat it with glucagon. 1 mg glucagon dose in adults may cause nausea or even vomiting with substantial, transient hyperglycemia. It has been shown that smaller doses (e.g., 150 mcg), repeated if necessary, were found to be effective in adolescents with T1DM without side effects [83]. The crystallized glucagon is diluted with the provided diluent to 1 mg/ml according to pharmaceutical instructions for the mini-dose regimen, and a U-100 insulin syringe is used to administer the dose [83]. Each unit on the U-100 insulin syringe represents ~10 µg of glucagon. For the dosing regimen, 2 "units" (20 µg) for children ≤2 years and 1 unit/year for children ≥3–15 years (with a maximum dose of 150 µg or "15 units") are advised to use. Older patients (young adults over 15 years of age) receive a maximum dose of 15 units (150 µg). If this dose does not increase blood glucose levels over the first 30 minutes, a repeat injection twice the initial dose should be done. An increase of 3.3–5 mmol/l in glucose levels is expected within 30 minutes of administration of the mini-dose glucagon regimen. The regimen is a safe and reliable tool to treat both mild and impending hypoglycemia in the out-of-hospital setting [83]. Liquid form and intranasal powder form of glucagon are other alternatives; however, there is limited data on the efficacy and safety of these glucagon preparations in treating hypoglycemia in the literature. A recent study by Suico et al. reported that nasal glucagon (3 mg) was as efficacious and well tolerated as intramuscular glucagon (1 mg) for the treatment of insulin-induced hypoglycemia in adults and will be as useful as intramuscular glucagon as a rescue treatment for SH [84]. Also, soluble glucagon and a glucagon analog, dasiglucagon, are available for immediate injection.

Patients with diabetes at increased risk of hypoglycemia are suggested to always carry glucagon with them. The relatives of patients should be educated about the administration of glucagon and the storage conditions of the agent. Apart from preventing severe hypoglycemia, it reduces emotional stress by means of empowering the patient's family and caregivers to take direct action and reduces medical care costs by avoiding the expensive use of emergency medical sources.

In glycogen-depleted individuals (e.g., following a binge of alcohol ingestion), glucagon may not be sufficient to increase glucose levels; 15–25 g intravenous glucose is the standard parenteral therapy initially. Because the response is transient, a subsequent intravenous glucose infusion may be needed, and a meal should be given to the patient as soon as the patient can eat.

4.3 Specific conditions

4.3.1 Management of nocturnal hypoglycemia

Apart from using insulin analogs to prevent nocturnal hypoglycemia, other approaches include bedtime snacks and bedtime administration of uncooked cornstarch for the sustained delivery of exogenous carbohydrates throughout the night. Bedtime oral administration of the epinephrine-stimulating ß2-adrenergic agonist terbutaline and overnight glucagon infusion may be other alternative treatments by providing sustained endogenous glucose throughout the night.

4.3.2 Management of exercise-induced hypoglycemia

Glucose consumption by the tissues increases during exercise with the risk of hypoglycemia. Strenuous, prolonged physical exercise with a lack of energy source is a great risk for hypoglycemia. To prevent hypoglycemia, blood glucose before and after physical exercise should be monitored. Patients should avoid injecting insulin to the part of the body that will be used during exercise because of increased blood flow to these body parts, resulting in faster insulin absorption during exercise, leading to hypoglycemia (e.g., injection insulin to the legs for running or cycling exercise). Moreover, time of exercise is important to prevent hypoglycemia. The consensus is to exercise in the postprandial period, but some studies show that exercising <45 min. When fasted, it results in stable blood glucose concentrations without the risk of hypoglycemia over the 24-hour post-exercise period [85]. Also, exercising in the morning is associated with a lower risk of hypoglycemia than exercising in the afternoon because of the high cortisol levels in the morning and low cortisol levels due to the circadian rhythm of cortisol. SH within the previous 24 hr. is a contraindication to do exercise, and if a self-treated hypoglycemic episode has occurred in the previous 24 hr., extra precautions should be taken before exercise, or it is better to avoid exercise alone. Prior to exercising, the blood glucose target should be >100 mg/dL. To minimize the hypoglycemia risk during and immediately following the exercise, additional carbohydrates (CHOs) prior to exercise may be needed. Patients are recommended to equip themselves with rapid-acting CHOs during physical exercise. This is called "ExCarb." A simple regimen is to take 30 g CHO every 60 min of exercise [86], or a more accurate method is to take CHO according to the body weight (0.5 gr/kg/h CHO for moderate-intensity activity and 1 gr/kg/h for high-intensity activity) [87]. Adjusting the insulin doses is also important to avoid hypoglycemia during exercise. Insulin pump therapy provides more flexibility for insulin adjustment. If an exercise is planned within 90 min after a meal, a 50% reduction should be made in the premeal insulin dosage. For insulin pump therapy users, the basal insulin dose should be reduced by 80% of the daily dose during the exercise period, starting 40 min before exercise and finishing at the end of the exercise. Late post-exercise hypoglycemia in T1DM typically occurs 6–15 hours after strenuous exercise and is usually nocturnal. **A** 50% reduction in the bolus dose given with the meal after the exercise and 20% reduction in the basal insulin at night reduces the risk of hypoglycemia. For patients with a history of recurrent hypoglycemia, the blood glucose should be checked at 02.00 h. In a recent study, a mini dose (150 μg) of glucagon was found to be more effective than reducing insulin dose to prevent exercise-induced hypoglycemia [88]. rt-CGM and flash glucose monitors are suggested to be used in case of exercise-induced hypoglycemia.

5. Conclusion

In summary, hypoglycemia in diabetes mellitus may result in anxiety and fear of subsequent events, leading to resistance to diabetes management. Severe hypoglycemia may cause cognitive dysfunction and seizures with an increased risk of cardiovascular disease and mortality. Taking measures to minimize the risk factors for the development of hypoglycemia and structured patient training is an important objective to prevent the occurrence of hypoglycemia in patients with T1DM. Advanced diabetes technologies such as CGMs, hybrid closed-loop pumps, and new insulins can be utilized. In contrast, widespread use of these systems is being hindered by cost-effectiveness, access, and education.

Author details

Kenan Sakar and Nese Cinar*
Faculty of Medicine, Department of Endocrinology and Metabolism Mugla, Mugla Sitki Kocman University, Turkey

*Address all correspondence to: cinarnese@gmail.com

References

[1] Patterson CC, Karuranga S, Salpea P, Saeedi P, Dahlquist G, Soltesz G, et al. Worldwide estimates of incidence, prevalence and mortality of type 1 diabetes in children and adolescents: Results from the International Diabetes Federation Diabetes Atlas. Diabetes Research and Clinical Practice. 2019;**157**:107842

[2] Vanderniet JA, Jenkins AJ, Donaghue KC. Epidemiology of type 1 diabetes. Current Cardiology Reports. 2022;**24**(10):1455-1465

[3] Januszewski AS, Cho YH, Joglekar MV, Farr RJ, Scott ES, Wong WK, et al. Insulin micro-secretion in type 1 diabetes and related microRNA profiles. Scientific Reports. 2021;**11**(1):11727

[4] Couper JJ, Haller MJ, Greenbaum CJ, Ziegler AG, Wherrett DK, Knip M, et al. ISPAD clinical practice consensus guidelines 2018: Stages of type 1 diabetes in children and adolescents. Pediatric Diabetes. 2018;**19**:20-27

[5] Mehers KL, Gillespie KM. The genetic basis for type 1 diabetes. British Medical Bulletin. 2008;**88**(1):115-129

[6] On behalf of the TEDDY Study Group, Lönnrot M, Lynch KF, Elding Larsson H, Lernmark Å, Rewers MJ, et al. Respiratory infections are temporally associated with initiation of type 1 diabetes autoimmunity: The TEDDY study. Diabetologia. 2017;**60**(10):1931-1940

[7] Yeung WCG, Rawlinson WD, Craig ME. Enterovirus infection and type 1 diabetes mellitus: Systematic review and meta-analysis of observational molecular studies. BMJ [Internet]. 2011;**342**:d35. Available from: https://www.bmj.com/content/342/bmj.d35.abstract [Accessed: November 21, 2023]

[8] Infante M, Ricordi C, Sanchez J, Clare-Salzler MJ, Padilla N, Fuenmayor V, et al. Influence of vitamin D on islet autoimmunity and beta-cell function in type 1 diabetes. Nutrients. 2019;**11**(9):2185

[9] Fourlanos S, Harrison LC, Colman PG. The accelerator hypothesis and increasing incidence of type 1 diabetes. Current Opinion in Endocrinology, Diabetes, and Obesity. 2008;**15**(4):321-325

[10] Uusitalo U, Lee HS, Andrén Aronsson C, Vehik K, Yang J, Hummel S, et al. Early infant diet and islet autoimmunity in the TEDDY study. Diabetes Care. 2018;**41**(3):522-530

[11] Agiostratidou G, Anhalt H, Ball D, Blonde L, Gourgari E, Harriman KN, et al. Standardizing clinically meaningful outcome measures beyond HbA1c for type 1 diabetes: A consensus report of the American Association of Clinical Endocrinologists, the American Association of Diabetes Educators, the American Diabetes Association, the Endocrine Society, JDRF international, the Leona M. and Harry B. Helmsley Charitable Trust, the pediatric Endocrine Society, and the T1D exchange. Diabetes Care. 2017;**40**(12):1622-1630

[12] Addendum CD. 11. Chronic kidney disease and risk management: Standards of medical care in diabetes—2022. Diabetes Care. 2022;**45**(Suppl. 1): S175-S184. Diabetes Care. 2022

[13] Nathan DM, Group DR. The diabetes control and complications trial/epidemiology of diabetes interventions and complications study at 30 years: Overview. Diabetes Care. 2014;**37**(1):9-16

[14] Elwen FR, Huskinson A, Clapham L, Bottomley MJ, Heller SR, James C, et al. An observational study of patient characteristics and mortality following hypoglycemia in the community. BMJ Open Diabetes Research & Care. 2015;**3**(1):e000094

[15] Pettus JH, Zhou FL, Shepherd L, Preblick R, Hunt PR, Paranjape S, et al. Incidences of severe hypoglycemia and diabetic ketoacidosis and prevalence of microvascular complications stratified by age and glycemic control in US adult patients with type 1 diabetes: A real-world study. Diabetes Care. 2019;**42**(12):2220-2227

[16] Skrivarhaug T, Bangstad HJ, Stene LC, Sandvik L, Hanssen KF, Joner G. Long-term mortality in a nationwide cohort of childhood-onset type 1 diabetic patients in Norway. Diabetologia. 2006;**49**:298-305

[17] Control D, Group CTR. Hypoglycemia in the diabetes control and complications trial. Diabetes. 1997;**46**(2):271-286

[18] Cherubini V, Pintaudi B, Rossi MC, Lucisano G, Pellegrini F, Chiumello G, et al. Severe hypoglycemia and ketoacidosis over one year in Italian pediatric population with type 1 diabetes mellitus: A multicenter retrospective observational study. Nutrition, Metabolism, and Cardiovascular Diseases. 2014;**24**(5):538-546

[19] Karges B, Rosenbauer J, Kapellen T, Wagner VM, Schober E, Karges W, et al. Hemoglobin A1c levels and risk of severe hypoglycemia in children and young adults with type 1 diabetes from Germany and Austria: A trend analysis in a cohort of 37,539 patients between 1995 and 2012. PLoS Medicine. 2014;**11**(10):e1001742

[20] Urakami T, Habu M, Suzuki J. Diabetic ketoacidosis and severe hypoglycemia in management of type 1 diabetes during 2003-2013. Pediatrics International. 2014;**56**(6):940-940

[21] Khunti K, Alsifri S, Aronson R, Cigrovski Berković M, Enters-Weijnen C, Forsén T, et al. Rates and predictors of hypoglycaemia in 27 585 people from 24 countries with insulin-treated type 1 and type 2 diabetes: The global HAT study. Diabetes, Obesity & Metabolism. 2016;**18**(9):907-915

[22] Lacy ME, Gilsanz P, Eng C, Beeri MS, Karter AJ, Whitmer RA. Severe hypoglycemia and cognitive function in older adults with type 1 diabetes: The study of longevity in diabetes (SOLID). Diabetes Care. 2020;**43**(3):541-548

[23] Amiel SA, Aschner P, Childs B, Cryer PE, de Galan BE, Frier BM, et al. Hypoglycaemia, cardiovascular disease, and mortality in diabetes: Epidemiology, pathogenesis, and management. The Lancet Diabetes and Endocrinology. 2019;7(5):385-396

[24] Vestergaard P, Rejnmark L, Mosekilde L. Relative fracture risk in patients with diabetes mellitus, and the impact of insulin and oral antidiabetic medication on relative fracture risk. Diabetologia. 2005;**48**:1292-1299

[25] Jensen MH, Vestergaard P. Hypoglycaemia and type 1 diabetes are associated with an increased risk of fractures. Osteoporosis International. 2019;**30**:1663-1670

[26] Johnson-Rabbett B, Seaquist ER. Hypoglycemia in diabetes: The dark side of diabetes treatment. A patient-centered review. Journal of Diabetes. 2019;**11**(9):711-718

[27] Rossi MC, Nicolucci A, Ozzello A, Gentile S, Aglialoro A, Chiambretti A, et al. Impact of severe and symptomatic

hypoglycemia on quality of life and fear of hypoglycemia in type 1 and type 2 diabetes. Results of the hypos-1 observational study. Nutrition, Metabolism, and Cardiovascular Diseases. 2019;**29**(7):736-743

[28] Dagogo-Jack S. Hypoglycemia in type 1 diabetes mellitus: Pathophysiology and prevention. Treatments in Endocrinology. 2004;**3**(2):91-103

[29] Pedersen-Bjergaard U, Agerholm-Larsen B, Pramming S, Hougaard P, Thorsteinsson B. Prediction of severe hypoglycaemia by angiotensin-converting enzyme activity and genotype in type 1 diabetes. Diabetologia. 2003;**46**:89-96

[30] Schouwenberg BJ, Coenen MJ, Paterson AD, Tack CJ, Smits P, Kramers C, et al. Genetic determinants of impaired awareness of hypoglycemia in type 1 diabetes. Pharmacogenetics and Genomics. 2017;**27**(9):323-328

[31] Cryer PE. Diverse causes of hypoglycemia-associated autonomic failure in diabetes. The New England Journal of Medicine. 2004;**350**(22):2272-2279

[32] Davis HA, Spanakis EK, Cryer PE, Davis SN. Hypoglycemia during Therapy of Diabetes. South Dartmouth (MA): MDText.com, Inc.; 2021

[33] Cryer PE, Davis SN, Shamoon H. Hypoglycemia in diabetes. Diabetes Care. 2003;**26**(6):1902-1912

[34] Banarer S, Cryer PE. Sleep-related hypoglycemia-associated autonomic failure in type 1 diabetes: Reduced awakening from sleep during hypoglycemia. Diabetes. 2003;**52**(5):1195-1203

[35] Cryer PE. Mechanisms of hypoglycemia-associated autonomic failure in diabetes. The New England Journal of Medicine. 2013;**369**(4):362-372

[36] Sanchez-Rangel E, Deajon-Jackson J, Hwang JJ. Pathophysiology and management of hypoglycemia in diabetes. Annals of the New York Academy of Sciences. 2022;**1518**(1):25-46

[37] Flatt AJ, Chen E, Peleckis AJ, Dalton-Bakes C, Nguyen HL, Collins HW, et al. Evaluation of clinical metrics for identifying defective physiologic responses to hypoglycemia in long-standing type 1 diabetes. Diabetes Technology & Therapeutics. 2022;**24**(10):737-748

[38] Nakhleh A, Shehadeh N. Hypoglycemia in diabetes: An update on pathophysiology, treatment, and prevention. World Journal of Diabetes. 2021;**12**(12):2036

[39] Sämann A, Mühlhauser I, Bender R, Kloos C, Müller UA. Glycaemic control and severe hypoglycaemia following training in flexible, intensive insulin therapy to enable dietary freedom in people with type 1 diabetes: A prospective implementation study. Diabetologia. 2005;**48**:1965-1970

[40] Plank J, Köhler G, Rakovac I, Semlitsch BM, Horvath K, Bock G, et al. Long-term evaluation of a structured outpatient education programme for intensified insulin therapy in patients with type 1 diabetes: A 12-year follow-up. Diabetologia. 2004;**47**:1370-1375

[41] Hopkins D, Lawrence IAN, Mansell P, Thompson G, Amiel S, Campbell M, et al. Improved biomedical and psychological outcomes 1 year after structured education in flexible insulin therapy for people with type 1 diabetes: The UK DAFNE experience. Diabetes Care. 2012;**35**(8):1638-1642

[42] Little SA, Leelarathna L, Walkinshaw E, Tan HK, Chapple O, Lubina-Solomon A, et al. Recovery

of hypoglycemia awareness in long-standing type 1 diabetes: A multicenter 2 × 2 factorial randomized controlled trial comparing insulin pump with multiple daily injections and continuous with conventional glucose self-monitoring (HypoCOMPaSS). Diabetes Care. 2014;**37**(8):2114-2122

[43] Blonde L, Umpierrez GE, McGill JB, Reddy SS, Berga SL, Bush M, et al. American Association of Clinical Endocrinology clinical practice guideline: Developing a diabetes mellitus comprehensive care plan—2022 update. Endocrine Practice. 2022;**28**(10):923-1049

[44] Hirsch IB. Insulin analogues. The New England Journal of Medicine. 2005;**352**(2):174-183

[45] Gough SC. A review of human and analogue insulin trials. Diabetes Research and Clinical Practice. 2007;**77**(1):1-15

[46] Pickup JC, Keen H, Parsons JA, Alberti KG. Continuous subcutaneous insulin infusion: An approach to achieving normoglycaemia. British Medical Journal. 1978;**1**(6107):204-207

[47] Bode BW, Johnson JA, Hyveled L, Tamer SC, Demissie M. Improved postprandial glycemic control with faster-acting insulin as part in patients with type 1 diabetes using continuous subcutaneous insulin infusion. Diabetes Technology & Therapeutics. 2017;**19**(1):25-33

[48] Malecki MT, Cao D, Liu R, Hardy T, Bode B, Bergenstal RM, et al. Ultra-rapid lispro improves postprandial glucose control and time in range in type 1 diabetes compared to lispro: PRONTO-T1D continuous glucose monitoring substudy. Diabetes Technology & Therapeutics. 2020;**22**(11):853-860

[49] Liu W, Yang X, Huang J. Efficacy and safety of insulin degludec versus insulin glargine: A systematic review and meta-analysis of fifteen clinical trials. International Journal of Endocrinology. 2018;**2018**:8726046

[50] Becker RH, Dahmen R, Bergmann K, Lehmann A, Jax T, Heise T. New insulin glargine 300 units·mL^{-1} provides a more even activity profile and prolonged glycemic control at steady state compared with insulin glargine 100 units·mL^{-1}. Diabetes Care. 2015;**38**(4):637-643

[51] Yeh HC, Brown TT, Maruthur N, Ranasinghe P, Berger Z, Suh YD, et al. Comparative effectiveness and safety of methods of insulin delivery and glucose monitoring for diabetes mellitus: A systematic review and meta-analysis. Annals of Internal Medicine. 2012;**157**(5):336-347

[52] Pickup JC, Sutton AJ. Severe hypoglycaemia and glycaemic control in type 1 diabetes: Meta-analysis of multiple daily insulin injections compared with continuous subcutaneous insulin infusion. Diabetic Medicine. 2008;**25**(7):765-774

[53] Group RS. Relative effectiveness of insulin pump treatment over multiple daily injections and structured education during flexible intensive insulin treatment for type 1 diabetes: Cluster randomised trial (REPOSE). BMJ. 2017;**356**:j1285

[54] Mastrototaro J. The MiniMed continuous glucose monitoring system (CGMS). Journal of Pediatric Endocrinology & Metabolism. 1999;**12**(13):751-758

[55] Brown SA, Kovatchev BP, Raghinaru D, Lum JW, Buckingham BA, Kudva YC, et al. Six-month randomized, multicenter trial of closed-loop control in

type 1 diabetes. The New England Journal of Medicine. 2019;**381**(18):1707-1717

[56] Tauschmann M, Allen JM, Wilinska ME, Thabit H, Stewart Z, Cheng P, et al. Day-and-night hybrid closed-loop insulin delivery in adolescents with type 1 diabetes: A free-living, randomized clinical trial. Diabetes Care. 2016;**39**(7):1168-1174

[57] Russell SJ, Hillard MA, Balliro C, Magyar KL, Selagamsetty R, Sinha M, et al. Day and night glycaemic control with a bionic pancreas versus conventional insulin pump therapy in preadolescent children with type 1 diabetes: A randomised crossover trial. The Lancet Diabetes and Endocrinology. 2016;**4**(3):233-243

[58] Russell SJ, El-Khatib FH, Sinha M, Magyar KL, McKeon K, Goergen LG, et al. Outpatient glycemic control with a bionic pancreas in type 1 diabetes. The New England Journal of Medicine. 2014;**371**(4):313-325

[59] Group JDRFCGMS. Continuous glucose monitoring and intensive treatment of type 1 diabetes. The New England Journal of Medicine. 2008;**359**(14):1464-1476

[60] Battelino T, Phillip M, Bratina N, Nimri R, Oskarsson P, Bolinder J. Effect of continuous glucose monitoring on hypoglycemia in type 1 diabetes. Diabetes Care. 2011;**34**(4):795-800

[61] Lind M, Polonsky W, Hirsch IB, Heise T, Bolinder J, Dahlqvist S, et al. Continuous glucose monitoring vs conventional therapy for glycemic control in adults with type 1 diabetes treated with multiple daily insulin injections: The GOLD randomized clinical trial. Journal of the American Medical Association. 2017;**317**(4):379-387

[62] Beck RW, Riddlesworth T, Ruedy K, Ahmann A, Bergenstal R, Haller S, et al. Effect of continuous glucose monitoring on glycemic control in adults with type 1 diabetes using insulin injections: The DIAMOND randomized clinical trial. Journal of the American Medical Association. 2017;**317**(4):371-378

[63] Bolinder J, Antuna R, Geelhoed-Duijvestijn P, Kröger J, Weitgasser R. Novel glucose-sensing technology and hypoglycaemia in type 1 diabetes: A multicentre, non-masked, randomised controlled trial. The Lancet. 2016;**388**(10057):2254-2263

[64] Beck RW, Hirsch IB, Laffel L, Tamborlane WV, Bode BW, Buckingham B, et al. The effect of continuous glucose monitoring in well-controlled type 1 diabetes. Diabetes Care. 2009;**32**(10):1378-1383

[65] van Beers CA, DeVries JH, Kleijer SJ, Smits MM, Geelhoed-Duijvestijn PH, Kramer MH, et al. Continuous glucose monitoring for patients with type 1 diabetes and impaired awareness of hypoglycaemia (IN CONTROL): A randomised, open-label, crossover trial. The Lancet Diabetes and Endocrinology. 2016;**4**(11):893-902

[66] Raccah D, Sulmont V, Reznik Y, Guerci B, Renard E, Hanaire H, et al. Incremental value of continuous glucose monitoring when starting pump therapy in patients with poorly controlled type 1 diabetes: The real trend study. Diabetes Care. 2009;**32**(12):2245-2250

[67] Bosi E, Choudhary P, De Valk HW, Lablanche S, Castañeda J, De Portu S, et al. Efficacy and safety of suspend-before-low insulin pump technology in hypoglycaemia-prone adults with type 1 diabetes (SMILE): An open-label randomised controlled trial. The Lancet Diabetes and Endocrinology. 2019;**7**(6):462-472

[68] Heinemann L, Freckmann G, Ehrmann D, Faber-Heinemann G, Guerra S, Waldenmaier D, et al. Real-time continuous glucose monitoring in adults with type 1 diabetes and impaired hypoglycaemia awareness or severe hypoglycaemia treated with multiple daily insulin injections (HypoDE): A multicentre, randomised controlled trial. The Lancet. 2018;**391**(10128):1367-1377

[69] Jensen MH, Vestergaard P, Hirsch IB, Hejlesen O. Use of personal continuous glucose monitoring device is associated with reduced risk of hypoglycemia in a 16-week clinical trial of people with type 1 diabetes using continuous subcutaneous insulin infusion. Journal of Diabetes Science and Technology. 2022;**16**(1):106-112

[70] Laffel LM, Kanapka LG, Beck RW, Bergamo K, Clements MA, Criego A, et al. Effect of continuous glucose monitoring on glycemic control in adolescents and young adults with type 1 diabetes: A randomized clinical trial. Journal of the American Medical Association. 2020;**323**(23):2388-2396

[71] Pratley RE, Kanapka LG, Rickels MR, Ahmann A, Aleppo G, Beck R, et al. Effect of continuous glucose monitoring on hypoglycemia in older adults with type 1 diabetes: A randomized clinical trial. Journal of the American Medical Association. 2020;**323**(23):2397-2406

[72] Zhang W, Liu Y, Sun B, Shen Y, Li M, Peng L, et al. Improved HbA1c and reduced glycaemic variability after 1-year intermittent use of flash glucose monitoring. Scientific Reports. 2021;**11**(1):23950

[73] Bergenstal RM, Tamborlane WV, Ahmann A, Buse JB, Dailey G, Davis SN, et al. Effectiveness of sensor-augmented insulin-pump therapy in type 1 diabetes. The New England Journal of Medicine. 2010;**363**(4):311-320

[74] Battelino T, Conget I, Olsen B, Schütz-Fuhrmann I, Hommel E, Hoogma R, et al. The use and efficacy of continuous glucose monitoring in type 1 diabetes treated with insulin pump therapy: A randomised controlled trial. Diabetologia. 2012;**55**:3155-3162

[75] Bergenstal RM, Klonoff DC, Garg SK, Bode BW, Meredith M, Slover RH, et al. Threshold-based insulin-pump interruption for reduction of hypoglycemia. The New England Journal of Medicine. 2013;**369**(3):224-232

[76] Ly TT, Nicholas JA, Retterath A, Lim EM, Davis EA, Jones TW. Effect of sensor-augmented insulin pump therapy and automated insulin suspension vs. standard insulin pump therapy on hypoglycemia in patients with type 1 diabetes: A randomized clinical trial. Journal of the American Medical Association. 2013;**310**(12):1240-1247

[77] Teo E, Hassan N, Tam W, Koh S. Effectiveness of continuous glucose monitoring in maintaining glycaemic control among people with type 1 diabetes mellitus: A systematic review of randomised controlled trials and meta-analysis. Diabetologia. 2022;**65**(4):604-619

[78] Maiorino MI, Signoriello S, Maio A, Chiodini P, Bellastella G, Scappaticcio L, et al. Effects of continuous glucose monitoring on metrics of glycemic control in diabetes: A systematic review with meta-analysis of randomized controlled trials. Diabetes Care. 2020;**43**(5):1146-1156

[79] Wang Y, Zou C, Na H, Zeng W, Li X. Effect of different glucose monitoring methods on bold glucose control: A systematic review and meta-analysis. Computational and Mathematical Methods in Medicine. 2022;**2022**:2851572

[80] Klak A, Manczak M, Owoc J, Olszewski R. Impact of

continuous glucose monitoring on improving emotional well-being among adults with type 1 diabetes mellitus: A systematic review and meta-analysis. Polish Archives of Internal Medicine. 2021;**131**(9):808-818

[81] Klonoff DC, Bergenstal RM, Garg SK, Bode BW, Meredith M, Slover RH, et al. ASPIRE in-home: Rationale, design, and methods of a study to evaluate the safety and efficacy of automatic insulin suspension for nocturnal hypoglycemia. Journal of Diabetes Science and Technology. 2013;**7**(4):1005-1010

[82] Hering BJ, Clarke WR, Bridges ND, Eggerman TL, Alejandro R, Bellin MD, et al. Phase 3 trial of transplantation of human islets in type 1 diabetes complicated by severe hypoglycemia. Diabetes Care. 2016;**39**(7):1230-1240

[83] Chung ST, Haymond MW. Minimizing morbidity of hypoglycemia in diabetes: A review of mini-dose glucagon. Journal of Diabetes Science and Technology. 2014;**9**(1):44-51

[84] Suico JG, Hövelmann U, Zhang S, Shen T, Bergman B, Sherr J, et al. Glucagon administration by nasal and intramuscular routes in adults with type 1 diabetes during insulin-induced hypoglycaemia: A randomised, open-label, crossover study. Diabetes Therapy. 2020;**11**:1591-1603

[85] Scott SN, Anderson L, Morton JP, Wagenmakers AJ, Riddell MC. Carbohydrate restriction in type 1 diabetes: A realistic therapy for improved glycaemic control and athletic performance? Nutrients. 2019;**11**(5):1022

[86] Gallen IW, Hume C, Lumb A. Fuelling the athlete with type 1 diabetes. Diabetes, Obesity & Metabolism. 2011;**13**(2):130-136

[87] Riddell MC, Gallen IW, Smart CE, Taplin CE, Adolfsson P, Lumb AN, et al. Exercise management in type 1 diabetes: A consensus statement. The Lancet Diabetes and Endocrinology. 2017;**5**(5):377-390

[88] Rickels MR, DuBose SN, Toschi E, Beck RW, Verdejo AS, Wolpert H, et al. Mini-dose glucagon as a novel approach to prevent exercise-induced hypoglycemia in type 1 diabetes. Diabetes Care. 2018;**41**(9):1909-1916

Chapter 3

Impact of the Use of Metformin in the Prevention of Gestational Diabetes Mellitus in the High-Risk Population: An Article Review

Enrique Valdés Rubio

Abstract

Gestational diabetes mellitus (GDM) is a condition characterized by a carbohydrate metabolism disorder of variable severity. The onset or first detection occurs during pregnancy. Its prevalence has increased dramatically in the last 10 years. Etiological factors that make these pregnant women a population at a high risk of developing GDM include maternal obesity, increase in maternal age, family history of diabetes mellitus, polycystic ovary (PCOS) and pregestational insulin resistance (PIR). The impact of metformin (MET), a second-generation insulin-sensitizing biguanide, on the prevention treatment of GDM has been studied with contradictory results. Through an article review of the literature, this chapter seeks to determine the safety and effectiveness of MET in preventing the development of GDM in patients with PIR in addition to evaluating the impact of oral hypoglycemic agents in the treatment of GDM and type 2 DM.

Keywords: gestational diabetes mellitus, insulin resistance, metformin, neonatal hypoglycemia, pregnancy, antidiabetic drug

1. Introduction

Insulin resistance (IR) [1–5] is a metabolic condition that is necessary for the growth and development of the fetus during its intrauterine life. As the pregnancy progresses, its severity increases, reaching its peak in the third trimester. However, a series of high perinatal risk pathologies may occur when IR exceeds the threshold of normality and/or when the concentration of its biomarkers is altered (adiponectin, leptin, SHBG and resistin) [6–9] such as spontaneous abortion, (GDM), hypertensive syndromes, prematurity, macrosomia, and hypoglycemia, etc. These effects are associated with a decrease in insulin sensitivity and low consumption of peripheral glucose with the purpose of ensuring the fetal energy source. When this balance is altered, GDM develops due to three different phenotypes: fasting hyperglycemia,

IntechOpen

postprandial hyperglycemia, and mixed hyperglycemia [5, 10, 11]. This condition is associated with fetal growth restriction (FGR) and preeclampsia (PE) as they have a common pathophysiological etiopathogenesis such as endothelial dysfunction, abnormal placentation, and/or a metabolically predisposing condition [9].

In this chapter, some clinical conditions linked to IR will be developed, and I will also further develop the conditions associated with PIR. More emphasis will be placed on the efficacy, safety and prophylactic impact of MET in preventing GDM, and I will comment on the adverse side effects of two hypoglycemic drugs which are used and that have been studied the most. Special emphasis will be made on one of the most important deleterious effects of these hypoglycemic agents: maternal-fetal hypoglycemia.

The prevalence of GDM has grown exponentially in our population, and this is based on the different glycemic cut-off points of the different international guidelines for making the diagnosis of GMD, so the prevalence varies between 9–16%. We know that GDM is defined when any type of carbohydrate intolerance that is diagnosed from the first trimester onwards in pregnancy is screened. When a GDM is diagnosed in ranges between 140 mg% and 200 mg%, the first line treatment is a change in lifestyle that includes a hypocaloric regimen, not less than 1500 calories per day, restricting carbohydrates (HDC), and aerobic physical activity. If there is no response after 2 weeks of treatment, insulin therapy is indicated, which is GOLD STANDARD.

In the last two decades, two drugs have been studied that have given hope to doctors and especially to mothers by not being repeatedly pricked and sometimes feeling the symptoms associated with INS. One is glyburide, a second-generation hypoglycemic agent, and metformin (MET), an insulinosensitizer, both are grouped in the group of oral hypoglycemic agents. Due to the pharmacokinetic characteristics and the minimal risk that the mother child binomial will be affected and as in the etiopathogenesis, there is a close relationship with insulin resistance. Due to some studies that highlighted the safety and efficacy as I will demonstrate later, I proposed to carry out a double-blind, randomized, case control, multicenter study to evaluate the prophylactic effect of MET in patients with pregestational insulin resistance (PIR) and secondarily the eventual protective effect in other high-risk perinatal pathologies, especially highlighting the potential risk of hypoglycemia in the mother-son binomial.

2. Methods

In this chapter, evidence will be provided related to the effectiveness and safety of the use of oral hypoglycemic agents (HPO) as alternatives to insulin (INS) in the prevention and treatment of GDM. Thus, the prescribed HPO must demonstrate good effectiveness when compared with insulin therapy, the gold standard in the treatment of GDM, and that it does not pose a risk to the health of the mother-child binomial. One of the most deleterious effects that the fetus could suffer is hypoglycemia, a side effect that will be developed described as follows.

A computerized search was performed in MEDLINE, PubMed and the Cochrane database to identify those studies that presented the following inclusion criteria: randomized controlled trials (RCT), meta-analyses, systematic reviews and methodologically correct studies that met the best standards of Evidence-Based Medicine, from 2010 to 2024. These studies investigated perinatal outcomes in women with a history of PIR who were treated prophylactically with MET and/or in women with GDM and whose results have evaluated mainly the presence of hypoglycemia.

The keywords used in the search were gestational diabetes mellitus, insulin resistance, metformin, neonatal hypoglycemia, pregnancy, antidiabetic drug.

The objective of this RCT study was to evaluate the prophylactic effect of MET in patients with pregestational insulin resistance (PIR) in the development of GDM and secondarily the eventual protective effect in other high-risk perinatal pathologies, especially highlighting the potential risk of hypoglycemia, in the mother-son-binomial. The objective of these studies was to compare perinatal outcomes among those treated with MET v/s INS. A total of 63 articles dealing with this topic were studied, of which 18 met the inclusion criteria requirement.

3. Definitions

Insulin resistance was defined by the presence of any of the following criteria: HOMA test greater than 2.5 and at least one of the following clinical conditions: polycystic ovary syndrome (PCOS), acrochordon and acanthosis. Parameters were suggested by the American Association of Clinical Endocrinologists and the American College of Endocrinologists [1–4].

The diagnosis of GDM was defined according to the criteria of the International Association of Diabetes and Pregnancy Study Groups Recommendations on the Diagnosis and Classifications of Hyperglycemia in Pregnancy or any type of Carbohydrate intolerance detected during pregnancy. This is diagnosed with a glucose tolerance test (OGTT), with a load of 75 grams, carried out between 24 and 26 weeks of gestation and in high-risk pregnant women at 32 weeks, with a fasting blood glucose greater than 105 mg/dl on two occasions or greater than 140 mg/dl at 2 hours [12].

On the other hand, the diagnosis of PE was defined as the presence of arterial hypertension associated with proteinuria in a pregnancy greater than 20 weeks and which is associated with the following findings: blood pressure of 140/90 mm/hg or more, repeated on two occasions separated by at least 6 hours, or a single blood pressure of 160/100 mmHg or more, associated with 24-hour proteinuria of 300 mg or more, in the absence of urinary tract infection [13].

Small for Gestational Age (SGA) was defined as a neonate with a weight less than the 10th percentile for their gestational age based on the local growth charts.

Large for Gestational Age (LGA) was defined as a neonate with a weight greater than the 90th percentile for to its gestational age based on the local growth charts.

Macrosomia is defined as a newborn weighing 4000 grams or more.

The perinatal outcomes that were studied included first trimester abortion, GDM, PE, fetal growth restriction (FGR), PP, maternal body mass index (BMI), newborn weight (NW), macrosomia, Cesarean section (CS) maternal and neonatal hypoglycemia and admission to the intensive care unit (NICU).

3.1 Deleterious effect of hypoglycemia on the mother-child binomial in fetal growth and development

It is important to highlight that glucose plays a fundamental role in providing the substrate to produce the energy that is needed for the synaptic transport of neurotransmitters [5, 14–16]. The brain is incapable of storing glucose, so even a slight interruption or decrease in its concentrations will interfere with the normal chemical signaling of the neurotransmitters [15]. Most studies show that there are no changes in heart rate or fetal movements during events of moderate maternal hypoglycemia. These findings suggest that the fetus can use alternative sources of energy (ketones and lactic acid) during these episodes [17].

One of the greatest concerns when indicating a hypoglycemic agent to a pregnant woman who has a degree of carbohydrate intolerance during pregnancy is the probable isolated or recurring hypoglycemia suffered by the mother-child pair. The severity of these hypoglycemias vary according to the hypoglycemic regimen used and that includes the three drugs that have been studied the most (INS, MET and GLI). Thus, severe hypoglycemia has been observed in up to 40% of pregnant women treated with INS and carriers of type 1 pregestational DM [14]. It is noteworthy that these episodes of hypoglycemia are recurrent and reach incidences of 22%. They are more frequent in the first trimester of pregnancy when the fetus is in the organogenesis stage [15, 17]. Despite the above, there is no clear evidence whether hypoglycemia plays an etiological role in embryopathies. However, studies on experimental animals exposed to recurrent hypoglycemia demonstrated an alteration in the weight of the offspring, with exaggerated weight gain or, failing that, insufficient weight [15]. Findings also observed in mothers exposed to recurrent hypoglycemia were observed in offspring. There was a higher incidence of macrosomia whose probable etiopathological explanation would be attributable to hyperglycemia reactive to hypoglycemia. In fact, the average HbA1c concentration of these patients was 5.6% [11]. It is rare for children of mothers who experience repetitive hypoglycemia to have permanent damage in their adult lives; however, studies are emerging that this recurrent exposure could be related to alterations in neurodevelopment, characterized by alterations in cognitive function and a greater risk of developing epilepsy [16, 17].

3.2 Physiological and protective role of insulin resistance during pregnancy and its etiopathogenic impact in the development of high-risk perinatal pathologies

IR is defined as a decreased cellular response to insulin stimulation. Its diagnosis is made through abnormal values of fasting insulinemia and/or homeostatic model assessment-insulin resistance HOMA-IR (>2.5) and at least one of the following clinical signs: acrochordons, acanthosis nigricans and polycystic ovary syndrome (PCOS) [1, 2]. It is related to various diseases and syndromes, especially in women, who have polycystic ovary syndrome (PCOS) [18, 19], diabetes mellitus type 2, metabolic syndrome and gestational diabetes mellitus (GDM). However, IR in pregnancy performs a fundamental function that consists of the release of Free Fatty Acids (FFA) [3], preferably metabolized by the mother, and maternal hyperglycemia that, through facilitated diffusion, produces fetal hyperglycemia, which is essential for the growth and development of the fetus. On the other hand, FFAs [3–5] catalyze pro-IR physiological mechanisms, forming a virtuous circle to generate energy. Although it is true that, at the beginning of pregnancy, IR is found in physiological levels, this situation increases in response to the hyperglycemic action of a series of hormones, among others: placental lactogen [3, 5], estrogens, progesterone and cortisol. As pregnancy progresses, IR increases, thus affecting the transcription and secretion of insulin from the beta cells of the pancreas. They fall into relative insulin insufficiency (INS), failing to manage a euglycemic environment and develop GDM, defined as any alteration of the carbohydrate metabolism diagnosed during pregnancy [12]. On the other hand, if this metabolic condition is associated with obesity and a sedentary lifestyle, the pathophysiological etiopathogenic mechanism of the disease increases in severity as a greater pro-inflammatory degree is associated.

The concentration of a series of biomarkers is altered such as resistin, adiponectin, SHBG and leptin [6–8]. These biomarkers have been studied by the author, with the hypothesis that the altered concentration of these mediators would be useful to evaluate the future risk of developing pregnancy diseases which include inflammation, endothelial dysfunction and abnormal placentation, typical factors described in the development of PE and FGR. Thus, I studied the behavior of the concentrations of adiponectin [8] and SHBG [9]. The result was that none of these cytokines were statistically significant in predicting PE and FRG when evaluated in the first trimester. However, when we studied whether PIR could play a role in the subsequent development of PE, we found that there was a predictive role [9].

Now, when we study the prominence of PIR defined with an altered HOMA-IR, signs suggestive of PCOS (acrochordon and acanthosis nigricans), polycystic-looking ovary, obesity as defined by the American and Association of Clinical Endocrinologists and American College of Endocrinologists [1, 2], we found a high association with the subsequent development of PE in the index group (8.4 v/s 4.2% $p < 0.05$), and the same occurred with GDM (9.2 v/s 2, 9%; $p < 0.005$) [9].

On the other hand, when the patient develops GDM and does not respond to the change in lifestyle as a first-line treatment, insulin therapy is prescribed which is considered the gold standard in the treatment of insulin-requiring pregnant women. In the last 25 years, numerous studies have been researched and published to clarify what the first-line treatment is in the therapy of GDM, and the results are still controversial.

In the first instance, based on methodologically flawed studies, the use of hypoglycemic agents was contraindicated, first-generation sulfonylureas, due to their high incidence of hypoglycemia and consequent fetal risk. Numerous studies began with the euglycemic capacity of glyburide, a second-generation sulfonylurea and hypoglycemic itself. Its pharmacokinetics made it attractive to study given that, at that time, it was believed that it was not metabolized by the placenta, and the mother-fetus exchange rate was equal to the fetus-mother exchange rate. Finally, it bound 99.8% to plasma proteins, which transformed it into a barrier for the fetus, preventing passage to the intrauterine environment and thus avoiding probable fetal hypoglycemia.

In 2000, Langer appeared co-publishing a study in the New England Journal of Medicine. He compared the effectiveness since those treated with glyburide reached euglycemia levels comparable to INS users (82 v/s 88%), respectively [20]. However, hypoglycemia was greater in the insulin group (41 v/s 4%, p0.003). Subsequently, a series of studies appeared that praised what was published by Langer, although there was always fear of the potential deleterious effect of fetal and/or neonatal hypoglycemia due to the intrinsic effect of glyburide. Afterwards, studies began to be published that highlighted a series of adverse effects in the newborn with the most important being hypoglycemia. One of the most conclusive studies is that of Camelo et al. [21], which despite being a retrospective study, compared the efficacy and safety of glyburide v/s insulin with devastating results: of the 110,879 pregnant women recruited, 9173 developed GDM, 8.3% were treated with glyburide ($n = 4982$) or insulin ($n = 4191$). Among the results, it was highlighted that: newborns of women treated with glyburide presented the following adverse effects a higher risk of being admitted to intensive care units. After adjusting for differences at baseline, newborns of women treated with glyburide ($RR = 1.41$; 95% CI, 1.23–1.62) had respiratory distress ($RR = 1.63$; 95% CI, 1.23–2.15), hypoglycemia ($RR = 1.40$; 95% CI, 1.00–1.95), birth injury ($RR = 1.35$; 95% CI, 1.00–1.82), and large for gestational age ($RR = 1.43$; 95% CI, 1.16–1.76) compared with those treated with insulin [21].

Soon, further research showed that glyburide crossed the placenta. Despite the risk of a sulfonylurea such as glyburide causing hypoglycemia, articles continued to be published with discouraging results. Thus, a meta-analysis [22] was published that included seven open studies, with 798 GD, and without data on the randomization method. Glyburide was associated with higher newborn weight, more macrosomia, with RR 2.62 (95% CI 1.35–5.08), and more neonatal hypoglycemia, RR 2.04 (95% CI 1.30–3.20). Overall drug failure was 6.37%. The frequency of maternal hypoglycemia was erratic. Only two studies compare glyburide with metformin, with statistically significant results favoring the use of MET with less macrosomia (RR 0.33) and fewer large infants for gestational age (RR 0.44) [23]. The failure rate in these studies was 26.8% for metformin and 23.5% for glyburide. All the data make it advisable not to use glyburide in the treatment of GD and type 2 DM.

Although it is true and despite the controversial results of glyburide, it is still being studied because a significant percentage achieved maternal metabolic objectives.

3.3 Metformin

The prominence of the genesis of IR in the etiopathogenesis of GDM and the insulin-sensitizing effect of MET, a second-generation biguanide, suggests that this drug could be of interest as a prophylactic and therapeutic treatment of GDM. If to the latter we add that the exposure of the fetus to MET is very low, with a placental partition coefficient of 36.3%, concentrations in cord blood of 0.1 to 2.9% mg/L and a renal clearance that becomes more potent as pregnancy progresses, it makes it ideal for treating high IR and could have excellent results in preventing and treating GDM [24]. However, as we will see later, exposure of the fetus to MET could present some deleterious fetal effects that are still controversial.

Numerous studies have been carried out which demonstrate that MET is equivalent and even superior to INS in achieving the proposed euglycemic objectives [24–27]. The problem is that the parameters for making the diagnosis of GDM vary between different centers. The same occurs when diagnosing pathological glycemia that informs us of hyper or hypoglycemia such as fasting glycemia, postprandial glycemia, HbA1c and random glycemia.

On the other hand, there are a variety of studies that support MET, concluding that it reduces the risk of neonatal hypoglycemia [24–27]. Although the cut-off points for making the diagnosis of hypoglycemia differed in the different studies, it was established that the thresholds of glycemia to make the diagnosis of neonatal hypoglycemia varied from <1.4 to <2.6 mmol/L. Although the study by Ainuddin could not confirm the protective effect of MET in pregnant women with type 2 DM, it did demonstrate a clear decrease in neonatal hypoglycemia when it was associated with INS (MET + INS: 7.8% to INS alone: 30%, $p < 0.001$) [28]. On the other hand, the MiTy study, which also studied pregnant women with type 2 DM, did not find significant differences in the incidence of neonatal hypoglycemia (RR O.82, 95% CI 0.52 TO 1.30) [29]. Lastly, a study drew a lot of attention as surprisingly the indication of monotherapy with MET was associated with a decrease in hypoglycemia; however, when this was associated with INS, the risk of neonatal hypoglycemia increased significantly [24].

The first positive effect of MET was the increase in fertility and the clear decrease in first trimester spontaneous abortions in PCOS patients [24]. But its greatest impact occurred when the MIG study was published with a sample number of 751 pregnant women with GDM and in which the biomedical results of the use of MET (373/751) v/s INS (378/751) published by Rowan were compared [25]. In this study, the following biomedical results presented by the MET user patients stood out: less weight gain, better glycemic control, fewer episodes of maternal and neonatal hypoglycemia. Two findings were unexpected, the first being that 46% of the MET user group had to be supplemented with INS and a high incidence of premature childbirth was observed ($P = 0.004$) [25].

The patients who required supplementation were those who had a higher body mass index (BMI > 30) ($p = 0.01$), high fasting blood glucose ($p < 0.001$), high HBa1c ($p < 0.001$), and a history of first trimester spontaneous abortion ($p < 0.001$), history of GDM in previous pregnancies and a greater number of multiparas ($p = 0.003$) [25].

On the other hand, another study whose objective was to evaluate the effectiveness of MET v/s INS in achieving euglycemic ranges in patients with type 2 DM, the results were disastrous, as 84.9% of the MET group had to be supplemented with INS [24]. Later, in 2020, the MiTy study was published in which 502 GDM participated. This study compared MET or placebo v/s INS, and among its results, the following was highlighted: the group treated with MET had lower HbA1c values, less maternal weight gain, lower incidence of cesarean section, lower weights of neonates (p.006), lower number of neonates classified as LGA (22 v/s 27%; p 0.041), but with a high incidence of SGA (13 v/s 7%, p0.026%) and greater chance of jaundice of the newborn (NB) [29].

Finally, a recent meta-analysis [28] that included six studies with 1362 treated with MET, confirmed less weight gain (−1.14 kg) and less pregnancy-induced hypertension with a relative risk (RR) of 0.53. A higher incidence of preterm birth was reported with RR 1.50 and a higher trend, but it did not reach a statistical significance of neonatal hypoglycemia. Adverse digestive effects varied between 2.5 and 45.7%, and gastro-intestinal intolerance forced the suspension of MET with an overall failure rate of 33.8% [28].

On the other hand, the proven transplacental passage and high fetal concentration of MET are cause for concern, and there is controversial information on the medium and long-term effects on children exposed intrauterinely to this drug. It can be concluded that metformin in GDM constitutes a therapeutic tool, achieving similar or even better glycemic concentrations than insulin in the NB in the short term, with better adherence to treatment and better control of maternal weight, but with the exception that preterm birth was more frequent and INS supplementation was necessary in more than a third of the cases. Digestive intolerance required suspension of its indication in around 30% [24].

No malformations were found and among the early and late effects in the offspring exposed to MET during pregnancy would be secondary to alteration in fetal programming, causing a greater predisposition to obesity during adolescence and metabolic syndrome in adulthood [24].

In another a study in which PCOS pregnant women were treated with MET during pregnancy, the follow-up of the exposed children presented higher fasting blood glucose and systolic blood pressure at 8 years of age [30]. Other study that researched children exposed to MET v/s INS concluded that, although weights were similar until 2 years of age, at 9 years of age, BMI was significantly higher in children exposed to MET (MD 0.98.95% CI o.23 to 1.33 $p = 0.005$) [31].

Finally, a systematic review and meta-analysis studied the impact on neurodevelopment in 7641 children up to 14 years of age, obtaining the following results: metformin use during pregnancy was not associated with neurodevelopmental delay in infancy (relative risk, 1.09; 95% confidence interval, 0.54e2.17; 3 studies; 9668 children) or at ages 3 to 5 years (relative risk, 0.90; 95% confidence interval, 0.56e1.45; 2 studies; 6118 children). When compared with unexposed peers, metformin use during pregnancy was not associated with altered motor scores (mean difference, 0.30; 95% confidence interval, 1.15 to 1.74; 3 studies; 714 children) or cognitive scores (mean difference, 0.45; 95% confidence interval, 1.45 to 0.55; 4 studies; 734 children), concluding that MET would not appear to affect neurodevelopment in children until age 14 [32].

Due to the aforementioned, some health agencies recommend its use as a first-line treatment in GDM, even though its indication is not explicitly authorized by the international drug control agencies.

Following these controversial results and based on the hypothesis that higher degrees of preconception IR would trigger GDM, I developed a hitherto unique, randomized, double-blind, multicenter study (RCT) of first-semester pregnant patients with the unique history of being only pregestational insulin resistance (PIR) carriers, with the objective of evaluating MET as a prophylactic treatment of GDM. For these objectives, two groups were created, one of them was prescribed 1700 mg of MET and the other placebo [33]. The diagnosis of pregestational PCOS was made with a history of fasting insulinemia greater than 15 uIU/l and/0 HOMA – IR greater than 2.5 and at least one of the following: acrochordon, acanthosis nigricans or the previous diagnosis of PCOS. It should be kept in mind that all the studies that have been carried out classifying them as PIR have been carried out on patients where IR may or may not be present and thus 70–80% of those patients who suffer from PCOS and obesity present IR. In thin women, it can be present between 30 and 40% [18, 19].

This study, which was carried out in 141 patients, was randomized (68 patients in the MTF group and 73 in the placebo group). The administration of MET was not associated with a decrease in GDM compared to placebo (37.5 v/s 25.4%, respectively; $P = 0.2$). On the other hand, the administered MET was associated with a high gastro-intestinal intolerance v/s placebo (14.3 v/s 1.8%, respectively; $P = 0.02$). Therefore, it can be concluded that MET is not effective as a GDM prophylaxis in patients with PIR [33].

A recent RCT study (EMPOWar) evaluated the potential prophylactic effect of MET in obese women (BMI = 30–39 KG/Mtr2 v/s BMI > 40 KG/Mtr2), to prevent high-risk perinatal pathologies, a population in which PIR does not always exist and who did not have type 2 DM at the time of recruitment [34]. A total of 449 women were randomized in the placebo group (n = 223) and in the MET group (n = 226) who were prescribed from 500 to 2500 mg/day. Various biomedical variables were analyzed in the mother and fetus, and in all the variables that were studied, no significant difference was found between the MET group and the placebo. The authors conclude that MET is not indicated in obese patients who do not present GDM. Therefore, the use of MET is not effective in the prevention of GDM in populations with PIR. The use of MTF shows a significantly higher frequency of drug intolerance than placebo [34].

Finally, based on multiple studies, they conclude that there is a group of patients with GDM who will present a poor response to MET and will probably need supplemental insulin therapy to achieve euglycemia [35–39].

4. Conclusions

MET presents evidence that supports its use in patients with GDM and even in patients suffering from type 2 DM, as it achieves similar metabolic objectives as INS, a decrease in first trimester spontaneous abortions in patients suffering from PCOS and could decrease in late pre-eclampsia in obese patients. Despite the latter, there are several methodologically valid studies that conclude the association of MET with a greater risk of premature birth and a notorious gastro-intestinal intolerance that causes its use to be suspended in one-third of the women under treatment. On the other hand, the use of MET has been shown to present early and late sequelae effects in those fetuses exposed to MET. Finally, the doses of MET proved to be indicated at random as IR increases during the course of pregnancy and its effect can take days. So, in patients who present pregestational type 2 DM, it must be accompanied by INS, as in the period of organogenesis where the fetuses can present severe and recurrent hypoglycemia, a deleterious and probably teratogenic effect that could leave early or late sequelae, which needs to be studied before suggesting it as a first-line treatment for type 2 DM or early GD. On the other hand, the use of MET would not have a prophylactic effect against developing GDM in patients with PIR. What is fairly clear is that the use of glyburide should be contraindicated throughout pregnancy.

Author details

Enrique Valdés Rubio
Fetal Medicine Unit, Department of Obstetrics and Gynecology, Hospital Clínico de la Universidad de Chile, Chile

*Address all correspondence to: e.valdes.r63@gmail.com

References

[1] Matthews DR, Hosker JP, Rudenski AS, Naylor BA, Treacher DF, Turner RC. Homeostasis model assessment: Insulin resistance and beta-cell function from fasting plasma glucose and insulin concentrations in man. Diabetologia. 1985;**28**:412-419

[2] Einhorn D, Reaven GM, Cobin RH, Ford E, Ganda OP, Handelsman Y, et al. American College of Endocrinology Position Statement on the insulin resistance syndrome. Endocrine Practice. 2003;**9**:237-252

[3] Sonagra AD, Biradar SM, Murthy DSJ. Normal pregnancy-a state of insulin resistance. Journal of Clinical and Diagnostic Research. 2014;**8**(11):CC01-CCC3

[4] Tumurbaatar B, Poole AT, Olson G, et al. Adipose tissue insulin resistance in gestational diabetes. Metabolic Syndrome and Related Disorders. 2017;**15**(2):86-92

[5] Reece EA, Homko C, Wiznitzer A. Metabolic changes in diabetic and nondiabetic subjects during pregnancy. Obstetrical & Gynecological Survey. 1994;**49**(1):64-71. DOI: 10.1097/00006254-199401000-00027

[6] D'Anna R, Baviera G, Corrado F, Giordano D, De Vivo A, Nicocia G, et al. Adiponectin and insulin resistance in early- and late-onset pre-eclampsia. BJOG. 2006;**113**:1264-1269

[7] Valdés ER, Lattes KA, Muñoz HS, Barja PY, Papapietro KV. First-trimester adiponectin and subsequent development of preeclampsia or fetal growth restriction. Gynecologic and Obstetric Investigation. 2011;**72**:152-156

[8] Valdés ER, Lattes KA, Muñoz HS, Cumsille M. Sex-hormone binding globulin (SHBG) levels dung pregnancy as predictors for pre-eclampsia and fetal growth restriction. Revista Médica de Chile. 2012;**140**:589-594

[9] Valdés E, Sepúlveda-Martínez A, Manukian B, Parra-Cordero M. Assessment of pregestational insulin resistance as a risk factor of preeclampsia. Gynecologic and Obstetric Investigation. 2014;**77**:111-116

[10] Plows JF, Stanley JL, Baker PN, Reynolds CM, Vickers MH. The pathophysiology of gestational diabetes mellitus. International Journal of Molecular Sciences. 2018;**19**(11):3342

[11] Moyce BL, Dolinsky VW. Maternal beta-cell adaptations in pregnancy and placental signalling: Implications for gestational diabetes. International Journal of Molecular Sciences. 2018;**19**(11):3467. DOI: 10.3390/ijms1911346

[12] International Association of Diabetes and Pregnancy Study Groups Consensus Panel, Metzger BE, Gabbe SG, et al. International Association of Diabetes and Pregnancy Study Groups recommendations on the diagnosis and classification of hyperglycemia in pregnancy. Diabetes Care. 2010;**33**:676-682

[13] American College of Obstetricians and Gynecologists. Gestational hypertension and preeclampsia: ACOG practice bulletin, No. 222. Obstetrics & Gynecology. 2020;**135**(6):e237-e260. DOI: 10.1097/AOG.0000000000003891

[14] Vadakekut ES. Association of maternal hypoglycemia with low birth weight and low placental weight: A retrospective investigation. The Journal of the American Osteopathic Association. 2011;**111**(3):148-152

[15] Pacaud D, Dewey D. Neurocognitive outcome of children exposed to severe hypoglycemia in utero. Review. Diabetes Management. 2011;**1**(1):129-140

[16] Di Ciannia G. Hypoglycemia in diabetic pregnancy front diabetes. Basel Karger. 2020;**28**:109-122

[17] Braak E et al. Maternal hypoglycemia during pregnancy in type 1 diabetes: Maternal and fetal consequences. Diabetes/Metabolism Research and Reviews. 2002;**18**:96-105

[18] Dumesic DA, Oberfield SE, Stener-Victorin E, Marshall JC, Laven JS, Legro RS. Scientific statement on the diagnostic criteria, epidemiology, pathophysiology, and molecular genetics of polycystic ovary syndrome. Endocrine Reviews. 2015;**36**:487-525

[19] Azziz R, Carmina E, Chen Z, Dunaif A, Laven JSE, Legro RS, et al. Polycystic ovary syndrome. Nature Reviews Disease Primers. 2016;**2**:16057

[20] Langer O, Conway DL, Berkus MD, et al. A comparsion of glyburide and insulin in women whit gestacional diabetes mellitus. The New England Journal of Medicine. 2000;**343**:1134

[21] Castillo WC, Boggess K, Stürmer T, Brookhart MA, Benjamin DK Jr, Funk MJ. Association of Adverse Pregnancy Outcomes with Glyburide vs insulin in women with gestational diabetes. JAMA Pediatrics. 2015;**169**(5):452-458. DOI: 10.1001/jamapediatrics.2015.74

[22] Guo L, Ma J, Tang J, Hu D, Zhang W, Zhao X. Comparative efficacy and safety of metformin, glyburide, and insulin in treating gestational diabetes mellitus: A meta-analysis. Journal Diabetes Research. 2019;**2019**:9084708. DOI: 10.1155/2019/9804708

[23] Balsells M, Garcia-Patterson A, Solá I, Roqué M, Corcoy R. Glibenclamide, metformin, and insulin for the treatment of gestational diabetes: A systematic review and meta-analysis. BMJ. 2015;**350**:h102. DOI: 10.1136/bmj.h102, (Published 21 January 2015)

[24] Tosti G, Barberio A, Tartaglione L, Rizzi A, Di Leo M, Viti L, et al. Lights and shadows on the use of metformin in pregnancy: From the preconception phase to breastfeeding and beyond. Frontiers in Endocrinology. 2023;**14**:1176623. DOI: 10.3389/fendo.2023.1270472. This article is part of the Research Topic Current and Future Trends in Gestational Diabetes Diagnosis and care

[25] Rowan JA, Hague WM, Gao W, Battin MR, Moore MP. Metformin versus insulin for the treatment of gestational diabetes. (MIG). The New England Journal of Medicine. 2008;**358**(19):2003-2015. DOI: 10.1056/NEJMoa0707193

[26] Stavroula A, Almog Shalit P, Gerontiti E, Kleoniki I, Theodoros A, Theodora K, et al. Efficacy and safety of metformin during pregnancy: An update. Endocrine. 2024;**83**:259-269

[27] Bao LX, Shi WT, Han YX. Metformin versus insulin for gestational diabetes: A systematic review and meta-analysis. The Journal of Maternal-Fetal & Neonatal Medicine. 2021;**34**(16):2741-2753

[28] Ainuddin JA, Karim N, Zaheer S, Ali SS, Hasan AA. Metformin treatment in type 2 diabetes in pregnancy: An active controlled, parallel-group, randomized, open label study in patients with type 2 diabetes in pregnancy. 2015. DOI: 10.1155/2015/32585

[29] Feig DS, Donovan LE, Zinman B, Sanchez JJ, Asztalos E, Ryan EA, et al. Metformin in women with type 2

diabetes in pregnancy (MiTy): A multicentre, international, randomised, placebo-controlled trial. The Lancet Diabetes and Endocrinology. 2020;**8**:834-844. DOI: 10.1016/S2213-8587(20)30310-70000004526

[30] Rø TB, Ludvigsen HV, Carlsen SM, Vanky E. Growth, body composition and metabolic profile of 8-year-old children exposed to metformin in utero. Scandinavian Journal of Clinical and Laboratory Investigation. 2012;**72**(7):570-575

[31] Brand KMG, Saarelainen L, Sonajalg J, Boutmy E, Foch C, Vääräsmäki M, et al. Metformin in pregnancy and risk of adverse long-term outcomes: A register-based cohort study. BMJ Open Diabetes Research & Care. 2022;**10**:2363. DOI: 10.1136/BMJDRC-2021-002363

[32] Gordon HG, Atkinson JA, Tong S, Mehdipour P, Cluver C, Walker SP, et al. Metformin in pregnancy and childhood neurodevelopmental outcomes: A systematic review and meta-analysis. American Journal of Obstetrics & Gynecology. 2024:S0002-9378(24)00430

[33] Valdés E, Sepúlveda-Martínez A, Candia P, Abusada N, Orellana R, Manukian B, et al. Metformin as a prophylactic treatment of gestational diabetes in pregnant patients with pregestational insulin resistance: A randomized study. The Journal of Obstetrics and Gynaecology Research. 2018;**44**(1):81-86

[34] Chiswick C, Reynolds RM, Denison F, Drake AJ, Forbes S, Newby DE, et al. Effect of metformin on maternal and fetal outcomes in obese pregnant women (EMPOWaR): A randomised, double-blind, placebo-controlled trial. The Lancet Diabetes and Endocrinology. 2015;**3**(10):778-786. DOI: 10.1016/S2213-8587(15)00219-3

[35] Spaulonci CP, Bernardes LS, Trindade TC, Zugain M, Francisco RP. Randomized trial of metformin vs insulin in the management of gestational diabetes. American Journal of Obstetrics and Gynecology. 2013;**209**(1):34.e1-34.e7

[36] Ashoush S, El-Said M, Fathi H, Abdelnaby M. Identification of metformin poor responders, requiring supplemental insulin, during randomization of metformin versus insulin for the control of gestational diabetes mellitus. The Journal of Obstetrics and Gynaecology Research. 2016;**42**(6):640-647

[37] Tertti K, Ekblad U, Koshinen P, Vahlberg T, Ronnemaa T. Metformin vs. insulin in gestational diabetes. A randomized study characterizing metformin patients needing additional insulin. Diabetes, Obesity & Metabolism. 2013;**15**(3):246-251

[38] Wong VW, Jalaludin B. Gestational diabetes mellitus: Who requires insulin therapy? The Australian & New Zealand Journal of Obstetrics & Gynaecology. 2011;**51**(5):432-436

[39] Gante I, Melo L, Dores J, Ruas L, Almeida M, do C. Metformin in gestational diabetes mellitus: Predictors of poor response. European Journal of Endocrinology. 2018;**178**(1):129-135

Chapter 4

Unveiling the Significance of the 'Bathtub' Shape in Blood Glucose Curve Analysis

Issa Rasheed Fetian

Abstract

Despite extensive research on insulin usage in diabetes, an effective method for regulating insulin dosage and timing has not emerged. Self-monitoring of blood glucose (SMBG) is crucial for diabetes self-care, but its utility is limited in intense insulin treatments. Moreover, persistent nighttime hypoglycaemia anxiety and neuropathic gastric issues pose significant challenges for patients with elevated nocturnal blood sugar and frequent post-meal hypoglycaemia. The "bathtub" curve outlines a daily glucose profile where levels spike after dinner, normalizing only after morning correction. This chapter focuses on addressing the difficulties posed by this glucose pattern for healthcare providers and researchers. The insights offered here could prove invaluable for diabetes management, potentially mitigating associated complications.

Keywords: insulin, hypoglycaemia, blood sugar profile, type 1 diabetes, self-monitoring of blood glucose (SMBG)

1. Introduction

Type 1 diabetes is a complex autoimmune disease characterized by the destruction of insulin-producing β-cells in the pancreas [1, 2]. This condition results in α-cell dysfunction, leading to reduced glucagon secretion during hypoglycemia. The delicate balance of blood glucose levels is maintained by a dynamic interplay of various factors, including insulin, glucagon, cortisol, adrenaline, and growth hormone [3]. Additionally, external factors such as stress, certain immunological processes, carbohydrate intake, and gluconeogenesis contribute to fluctuations in blood glucose levels. Furthermore, the role of weight management in influencing insulin action cannot be understated [4]. In this complex landscape of diabetes management, Self-Monitoring of Blood Glucose (SMBG) emerges as a crucial tool. SMBG provides immediate feedback on blood glucose levels, allowing individuals to make informed decisions about their insulin dosages, dietary choices, and physical activity. Regular SMBG, combined with appropriate adjustments in insulin therapy, diet, and lifestyle, can lead to improved long-term glycemic control, as reflected in lower hemoglobin A1c (HbA1c) levels [5]. Beyond these advantages, SMBG empowers individuals with type 1 diabetes to take an active role in their self-care and fosters a deeper understanding of how various factors affect blood glucose levels.

The regulation of glucose homeostasis is a multifaceted process influenced by circadian rhythms, which affect insulin sensitivity throughout the day [6]. Moreover, physical activity and the body's natural insulin secretion also play significant roles in lowering blood glucose levels [7]. Given the potential for insulin to induce acute severe hypoglycemia and the cardiovascular complications associated with elevated blood glucose, there is a paramount need to strive for "near normoglycemia."

Managing type 1 diabetes is an intricate and ongoing challenge, necessitating a continuous balancing act [5, 8–10]. To address these complexities and improve patient outcomes, individuals with type 1 diabetes must learn to manipulate many of these factors. This manipulation often involves the application of external subcutaneous insulin and diligent self-monitoring of blood glucose levels. Therefore, understanding the intricate web of factors that influence glucose homeostasis is essential for effective diabetes management. In this context, this article aims to delve deeper into the multifaceted nature of type 1 diabetes, shedding light on the various factors involved and the challenges faced by those living with the condition.

2. Clinical insights and observations

In 2022, we were motivated to publish a case report pertaining to this chapter, where we provided an in-depth analysis of the details. In the discussion section, we delve further into the specifics of our findings [11].

Since the pancreas transplant rejection [12], the patient has benefited from continuous subcutaneous glucose monitoring with programmable alarm thresholds, which trigger pre-emptive alerts for decreasing or increasing blood sugar levels. However, persistent nocturnal hypoglycaemic anxiety and neuropathic-induced gastric paresis remained significant challenges. These were associated with elevated nocturnal blood sugar levels and frequent postprandial hypoglycaemic episodes. Hypoglycaemic events lead to high blood sugar levels hours later due to excessive carbohydrate intake and prolonged counter-regulatory responses of insulin antagonists such as adrenaline, cortisol, glucagon, and growth hormone. Prolonged type 1 diabetes can disrupt this counter-regulation, often resulting in a lack of surge in adrenaline and glucagon during hypoglycaemia. Hypoglycaemia significantly contributes to the development of long-term complications in type 1 diabetes patients, particularly through excessive carbohydrate consumption following hypoglycaemic episodes [13]. In our previous publication [11] related to the mentioned patient, this occasionally led to the paradoxical situation where reducing insulin resulted in partial improvement of HbA1c levels.

The so-called "bathtub" curve describes a blood glucose daily profile in which blood sugar levels rise after dinner and only return to the target range after waking up in the morning [14]. The primary cause of such a pattern is the challenging-to-treat nocturnal hypoglycaemic anxiety experienced by patients. After dinner, blood sugar is intentionally kept above the target range, achieved either by administering less prandial insulin than necessary or by consuming a small snack before sleep. The goal is to avoid nocturnal hypoglycaemia, to which one is vulnerable while asleep. Hypoglycaemic anxiety is common in type 1 diabetes and plays a significant role in patients whose blood sugar levels are not satisfactorily manageable [15].

To address this issue, particularly in the first years following diagnosis until sufficient experience in everyday insulin management is gained, special attention should be given to avoiding severe hypoglycaemic episodes. To prevent this situation, diabetologists generally set slightly higher target blood sugar levels during the initial phase of insulin therapy. Once hypoglycaemic anxiety develops, it becomes challenging to treat, often persisting throughout the patients' lives. This is particularly concerning, given that the night constitutes about one-third of one's lifetime and contributes significantly to the development of complications.

In this scenario, prolonged inadequate blood sugar control with correspondingly high HbA1c levels led to neuropathic gastric paresis. This condition further contributes to the "bathtub" shape of the blood glucose daily profile, as food, and consequently the ingested carbohydrates, remain in the stomach for a longer duration. They are only gradually passed from the stomach to the intestines for absorption, primarily occurring in the evening. For the patient, this resulted in a delayed increase in blood sugar levels, often occurring many hours after a meal. Consequently, the gastric paresis led to early postprandial hypoglycaemic episodes due to rapidly acting insulin shortly after eating. This exacerbates daytime hypoglycaemic issues and is further intensified by attempts to compensate for intentionally elevated nighttime blood sugar levels by maintaining values near the hypoglycaemic threshold during the day.

In terms of differential diagnosis, changes in insulin requirements and consequent additional blood glucose fluctuations must also consider conditions such as thyroid dysfunction (generally yielding slightly higher blood glucose levels), adrenal insufficiency (reduced insulin requirement, leading to hypoglycaemia primarily at night), or celiac disease (carbohydrate malabsorption). All these disorders occur within the context of a polyglandular autoimmune syndrome, with a lifetime prevalence of approximately 15–30%, more frequently observed in type 1 diabetes mellitus [16]. Throughout the years of care, these conditions were repeatedly ruled out in the patient's case.

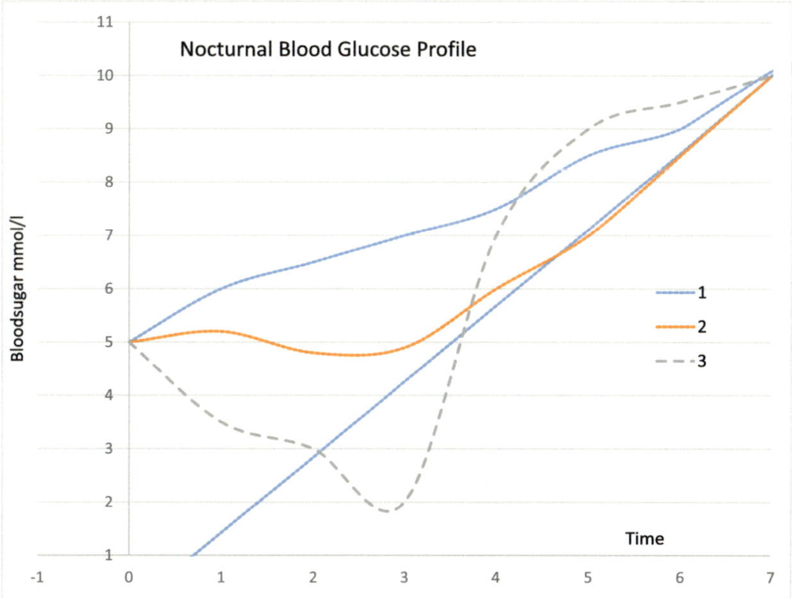

Figure 1.
Nocturnal blood glucose (BG) profile: differential diagnosis: high BG in the morning with normal BG before bedtime. The curve represents average values at the same times of day over a fixed period. 1. Insufficient basal insulin during the night; 2. Dawn phenomenon (marked circadian rhythm with an early-morning rise in BG); 3. Excessive glucose intake after hypoglycemia.

The patient's blood glucose trajectory is depicted in **Figure 1**. The dose of basal insulin should primarily be determined based on the metabolism of glucose, which mainly originates from liver production during the night. On the other hand, rapid-acting insulin should be adjusted mainly according to the quantity of orally ingested carbohydrates during the daytime. Since usually no food is consumed at night, having an identical blood glucose level at "bedtime" (blood glucose measured just before sleeping) and in the morning upon waking indicates that basal insulin was appropriately dosed for the night, regardless of whether both values are high or normal. This is also reflected in a bathtub curve. Therefore, comparing "bedtime" blood glucose to morning levels is a crucial aspect in evaluating blood glucose profiles.

A nearly physiological ratio of basal insulin to total insulin ranging from 30 to 50% is also indicative of optimal basal insulin dosing. Often, individuals with type 1 diabetes themselves limit their daily carbohydrate intake to reduce the dose of rapid-acting insulin, consequently increasing the percentage of basal insulin (as was the case with the described patient, reaching 60%).

Sometimes, it can be challenging to estimate the appropriate proportion of basal insulin, especially when rapid-acting correction insulin (as a replacement for basal insulin) is used for higher blood glucose levels regardless of meals. A so-called "meal omission test" can be helpful: if blood glucose remains stable during the test, it can be assumed that the basal rate is set correctly. In the case of the described patient, who regularly conducted such tests, the basal rate was usually set accurately.

When the "bedtime" blood glucose is within the target range, but the morning blood glucose is elevated, three classic differential diagnoses should be considered (**Figure 2**). These differential diagnoses can be distinguished through an analysis of the overnight blood glucose measurements:

1. Excessive carbohydrate intake after nocturnal hypoglycaemia. The previously described Somogyi effect, which explained a counter-regulatory response with elevated morning blood glucose following nighttime hypoglycaemia, can lead to a similar profile. However, this effect is currently considered scientifically questionable to non-existent and is deemed highly unlikely due to the impaired adrenergic counter-regulation in long-standing type 1 diabetes. More often, the cause is excessive carbohydrate intake [17].

2. Insufficient basal insulin to cover hepatic glucose output during the night: continuous rise in blood glucose from the "bedtime" measurement until early morning; subsequently, regular elevated blood glucose levels in the morning, if the liver's glycogen reservoir was sufficiently replenished with carbohydrates consumed orally during the day.

3. Dawn or sunrise phenomenon [18]: blood glucose level around 3 AM is identical to the "bedtime" reading; then there is a subsequent increase in blood glucose levels towards the morning; this can be explained by the circadian rhythm of endogenous insulin antagonists (such as adrenaline, growth hormone, glucagon, and cortisol).

Throughout the diabetes journey, such patients intentionally used insufficient basal insulin despite having hypoglycemic anxiety, even though their blood glucose levels were within the "bedtime" target range. A pronounced dawn phenomenon, which can also occur due to an innate circadian rhythm variation, was not present.

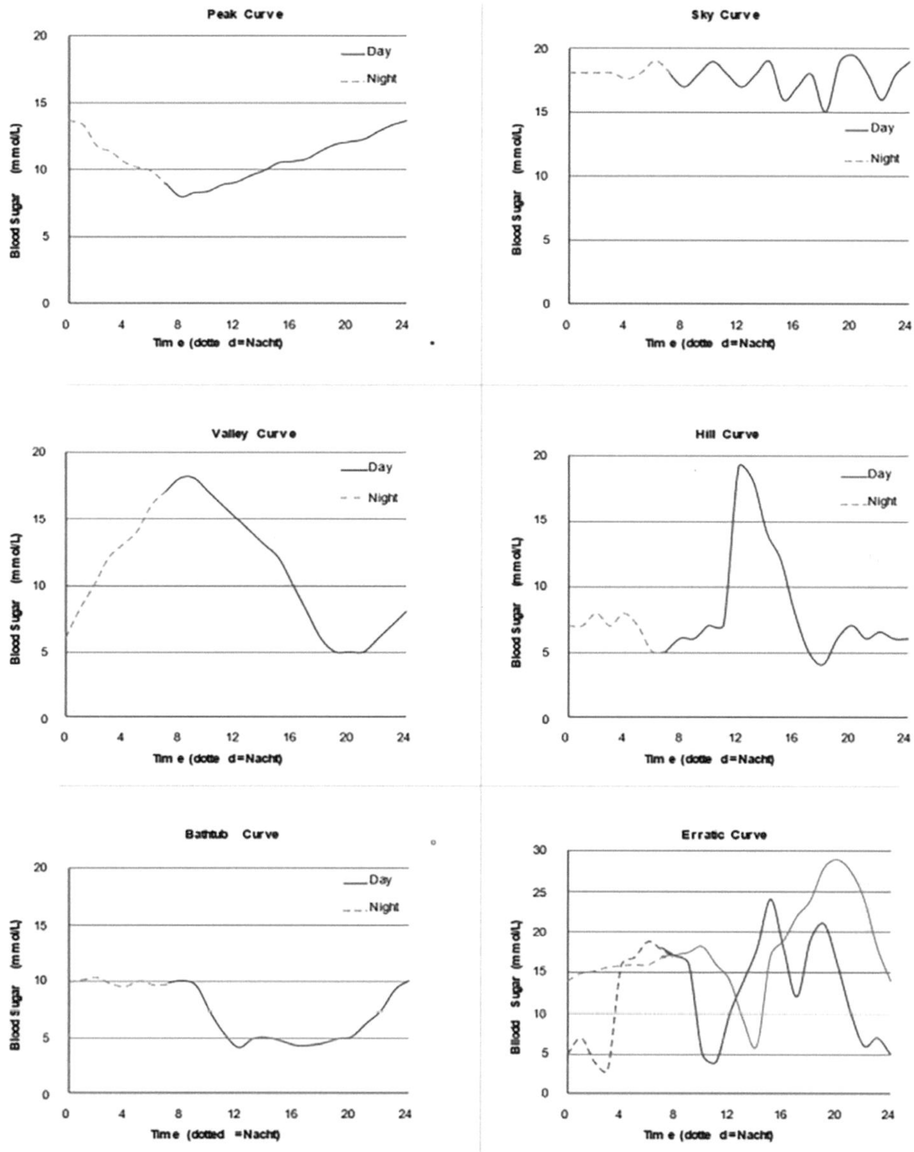

Figure 2.
Typical blood glucose daily profiles: model theoretical representation. Explanation and most common causes, see ***Table 1****. Adapted from Fetian et al. [11].*

Other reasons that contributed to increased blood glucose fluctuations and accentuated the risk of nocturnal hypoglycemia during the course of the patient's diabetes journey were:

Theoretical model representation, see **Figure 2**.

1. Under the immunosuppressive corticosteroid therapy following the pancreas transplant, daytime blood glucose levels increased due to the stimulation of

gluconeogenesis in the liver. Consequently, this led to nocturnal hypoglycemia as a result of the liver's depleted glucose reservoir.

2. The developing renal insufficiency necessitated a gradual reduction in insulin dosage for the patient due to the diminished breakdown of insulin, which occurs to about one-third through renal pathways.

3. In addition to the mentioned "bathtub curve," there are various other blood glucose daily profile patterns well-known to diabetologists, such as the peak, valley, hill, sky, or erratic (unpredictable) blood glucose curve. In **Figure 2** and **Table 1**, the manifestation and causes of these daily profiles are theoretically summarized. Over the course of her illness, the patient experienced each of these characteristic curve patterns repeatedly.

The long-term care of patients with type 1 diabetes requires a significant amount of experience and interdisciplinary collaboration. Patients with type 1 diabetes frequently encounter new situations that demand flexible and differentiated responses. In addition to well-established and often non-textbook knowledge (such as the reasons leading to typical blood glucose daily profiles, often conveyed by experienced diabetologists), patients should also be continuously offered the latest technological aids.

The presented case illustration depicted an extreme course of type 1 diabetes, through which many situations that diabetologists regularly encounter were described. When patients receive appropriate training from the outset of type 1 diabetes diagnosis, they often have a good chance of managing the condition effectively

Name of the theoretical model of the blood glucose curve	**Description of blood glucose**	**Most common causes of blood glucose curves in type 1 diabetes with 3 main meals and basal/bolus insulin**
Peak	Increasing over the day, decreasing at night	Excessive basal insulin at night, carbohydrate/insulin imbalance during all meals throughout the day
Sky	All blood glucose values high	Insufficient daytime insulin, as there is no overnight rise in blood glucose levels, the basal insulin is at least sufficient during the night
Valley	Decreasing over the day and gradually increasing over the night	Insufficient basal insulin at night, morning bolus insulin for not yet optimally achieved postprandial target values
Hill	Short-term blood glucose increase	Inadequate bolus insulin relative to carbohydrates during a meal
Bathtub	Higher at night compared to daytime.	Carbohydrate/insulin imbalance during dinner
Erratic	Unpredictable, constantly changing blood glucose values (blue day 1/yellow day 2)	Insulin-carbohydrate ratio rarely adjusted or lipodystrophies causing irregular subcutaneous insulin absorption or lack of adjustment for intense physical activity

Table 1.
Explanation and most common causes for typical blood glucose daily profiles.

in their daily lives. This can help maintain their quality of life and significantly reduce the risk of a shortened lifespan [11]. Overall, such dramatic courses, involving nearly all conceivable complications as in the present case, remain exceptions.

The patient demonstrated remarkable perseverance, never giving up and continuously striving to manage her "brittle diabetes."

3. Conclusion

Type 1 diabetes patients experience a wide array of blood glucose profiles throughout the course of their illness. The underlying causes are often ambiguous and diverse, influenced by factors such as dietary habits, physical activity, improper handling of technology, side effects of insulin therapy or other treatments, comorbidities, and stress. Occasionally, blood glucose profiles can be quite suggestive, as seen in intentionally accepted high nighttime blood glucose levels due to hypoglycemic fear, resulting in a "bathtub curve" (elevated blood glucose in the morning and at "bedtime," but normal during the day). The assessment of blood glucose profiles is central to the education and care of patients with type 1 diabetes.

The case demonstrates that even experienced diabetologists find that the existing tools of insulin therapy might not suffice to avoid such blood glucose daily profiles. However, it is hopeful that the planned "semi-closed-loop" insulin therapy for the patient will significantly improve blood glucose levels.

4. Summary

Blood glucose daily profiles of patients with diabetes are of paramount importance for better disease management and continue to pose a challenge for diabetologists. In the present case of a patient with long-standing type 1 diabetes and severe complications, a characteristic "bathtub" profile of the blood glucose curve is showcased. This specific pattern stems from the patient's behavior driven by nocturnal hypoglycaemic fear. The patient intentionally allows her blood glucose to rise after dinner until the morning, only lowering the blood glucose levels after waking up the next morning. Through this example, differential diagnostic considerations for various commonly occurring blood glucose daily profile patterns are discussed.

Acknowledgements

I extend my sincere appreciation to Dr Lukas Villiger for his invaluable support in endocrinology and to my dedicated team at HAP MZB for their collaboration. I'm grateful to Prof. Josef Flammer whose passion for science and commitment to excellence have been a constant source of inspiring me.

I would like to acknowledge Healthbook Times for their collaboration, as the adapted figure was generously provided by H+O Communications Ltd., Zurich, Switzerland. Their contribution greatly enhanced the quality of this work.

I am deeply indebted to my beloved uncle, Dr. Issa Fitian, my brother Ashraf Fetian, my mother, my wife, my daughter, and the rest of my family for their unwavering encouragement and belief in my pursuits. Their support has been a pillar of strength throughout this endeavour.

Last but not least, I extend my deepest gratitude to Palestine, my homeland, and express profound respect for the spirits of the Palestinian community, particularly the courageous doctors whose inspiration drives our advancements in the field of medicine.

Funding

This work received no specific grant from any funding agency in the public, commercial, or non-profit sectors.

Conflicts of interest

The author declare that there are no commercial or financial relationships that could be construed as potential conflicts of interest.

Author details

Issa Rasheed Fetian[1,2]

1 General Internal Medicine, Hausarztpraxis MZ-Brugg and DiaMon Institut, Brugg, Switzerland

2 University of Basel, Switzerland

*Address all correspondence to: irfetian@protonmail.com; issa.fetian@gmail.com

References

[1] Rodriguez-Calvo T, Ekwall O, Amirian N, Zapardiel-Gonzalo J, von Herrath MG. Increased immune cell infiltration of the exocrine pancreas: A possible contribution to the pathogenesis of type 1 diabetes. Diabetes. 2014;**63**(11):3880-3890. Available from: https://www.ncbi.nlm.nih.gov/pmc/articles/PMC4207385/

[2] Yosten GLC. Alpha cell dysfunction in type 1 diabetes. Peptides. 2018;**100**:54-60

[3] Lager I. The insulin-antagonistic effect of the counterregulatory hormones. Journal of Internal Medicine Supplement. 1991;**735**:41-47. Available from: https://pubmed.ncbi.nlm.nih.gov/2043222/

[4] Algoblan A, Alalfi M, Khan M. Mechanism linking diabetes mellitus and obesity. Diabetes, Metabolic Syndrome and Obesity: Targets and Therapy. 2014;**7**:587-591. Available from: https://www.ncbi.nlm.nih.gov/pmc/articles/PMC4259868/

[5] Cryer PE. Hypoglycemiais the limiting factor in the management of diabetes. Diabetes/Metabolism Research and Reviews. 1999;**15**(1):42-46

[6] Poggiogalle E, Jamshed H, Peterson CM. Circadian regulation of glucose, lipid, and energy metabolism in humans. Metabolism. 2018;**84**:11-27. Available from: https://www.metabolismjournal.com/article/S0026-0495(17)30329-3/abstract

[7] Riddell M, Perkins BA. Exercise and glucose metabolism in persons with diabetes mellitus: Perspectives on the role for continuous glucose monitoring. Journal of Diabetes Science and Technology. 2009;**3**(4):914-923

[8] Unger RH, Orci L. Paracrinology of islets and the paracrinopathy of diabetes. Proceedings of the National Academy of Sciences. 2010;**107**(37):16009-16012

[9] Cryer P. Hypoglycaemia: The limiting factor in the glycaemic management of Type I and Type II Diabetes*. Diabetologia. 2002;**45**(7):937-948

[10] American diabetes association. Standards of Medical Care in Diabetes—2022 abridged for primary care providers. Clinical Diabetes. 2022;**40**(1). Available from: https://diabetesjournals.org/clinical/article/40/1/10/139035/Standards-of-Medical-Care-in-Diabetes-2022

[11] Fetian IR, Maziukas R, Pisarcikova Z, Zechmann S, Dolinar M, Dolinar S, et al. "Bathtub" shape is a key term for interpreting the course of blood glucose curves. Healthbook TIMES Das Schweizer Ärztejournal Journal Des Médecins Suisses. 2022;**5**(1-2):98-104. Available from: https://schw-aerztej.healthbooktimes.org/article/34250-bathtub-shape-is-a-key-term-for-interpreting-the-course-of-blood-glucose-curves

[12] Weinzimer SA, Steil GM, Swan KL, Dziura J, Kurtz N, Tamborlane WV. Fully automated closed-loop insulin delivery versus semiautomated hybrid control in Pediatric patients with type 1 diabetes using an artificial pancreas. Diabetes Care. 2008;**31**(5):934-939

[13] The Diabetes Control and Complications Trial Research Group. Hypoglycemia in the diabetes control and complications Trial. Diabetes. 1997;**46**(2):271-286

[14] Suh S, Kim JH. Glycemic variability: How do we measure it and why is it

important? Diabetes & Metabolism Journal. 2015;**39**(4):273. Available from: https://www.ncbi.nlm.nih.gov/pmc/articles/PMC4543190/

[15] Brod M, Pohlman B, Wolden M, Christensen T. Non-severe nocturnal hypoglycemic events: Experience and impacts on patient functioning and well-being. Quality of Life Research. 2012;**22**(5):997-1004

[16] Komminoth P. Polyglanduläre autoimmune Syndrome. Der Pathologe. 2016;**37**(3):253-257

[17] Gale EAM, Kurtz AB, Tattersall RB. In search of the Somogyi effect. The Lancet. 1980;**316**(8189):279-282

[18] Carroll MF, Schade DS. The Dawn phenomenon revisited: Implications for diabetes therapy. Endocrine Practice. 2005;**11**(1):55-64

Chapter 5

Estimation of HbA1c and Impact of Continuous Glucose Monitoring in Hypoglycemic States

Brijesh Kumar Mishra, Alok Raghav, Goo-Bo Jeong, Mukesh Jain, Pinky Shukla and Swati Sharma

Abstract

Glycosylated hemoglobin (HbA1c) is formed when glucose combines with hemoglobin present in red blood cells making it glycated. Hypoglycemia is presented by less sugar binding with the hemoglobin compared to in hyperglycemia. HbA1c is considered to be a gold standard for measuring glycemic index in diabetic patients. This indicates the burden of blood glucose in subjects with diabetes mellitus. As the normal life span of red blood cells (RBCs) is 90–120 days, therefore HbA1c predicts the average glucose level of 90 days period. Currently, it is being used to combat the burden of diabetes worldwide. There are several cost-effective and high sensitivity & specificity techniques that are being used for the measurement of HbA1c. Most advanced methods include HPLC and enzyme-based. However, there are some variants of hemoglobin that interfere with it. As this is one of the essential parameters to study the progression of diabetes in a patient, a cost-effective and reliable method is required for the estimation.

Keywords: glycosylated hemoglobin, diabetes mellitus, hypoglycemia, quantification, HbA1c

1. Introduction

The overall burden of type 2 diabetes mellitus has a rising trend in the world. The global prevalence of diabetes among the general population was estimated at 150 million in 1995, which is projected to increase to 300 million by 2025 [1, 2]. Management of glycemia in diabetes patients is the need of the hour. Hemoglobin A1c (HbA_1c) or glycated hemoglobin (GHB) is a diagnostic biomarker that is extensively used routinely worldwide in the management of individuals with glucose intolerance to monitor long-term glycemic control and to assess the risk of developing complications. HbA_1c is the advanced product of glycosylation reaction between sugar and protein that is very stable and is almost unaffected by the fluctuation of blood glucose. Currently, it is recognized as the gold standard for long-term glycemic control. HbA_1c was discovered in the late 1960s by Samuel Rahbar, as a fast-moving hemoglobin in diabetic patients. He reported that two diabetic patients out of 1200 subjects had an abnormal fast-moving hemoglobin fraction [3]. Bookchin and Gallop confirm their structure while separating hemoglobin fragments that had a hexose moiety linked to the N-terminus of the f3-globin chain. Later, Anthony Cerami also contributed to the development of HbA1c as a clinical marker. This breakthrough came in 1968 and was not immediately appreciated broadly. Its use as a marker of glycemic control has gradually increased over the last four decades [4]. The American Diabetes Association (ADA) acknowledged the work of Rahbar in the year 2012, and in past decades, HbA1c gained attention as gold standard for screening of glycemic control, making it a convenient method for both doctor and patient, for the first time, to critically assess the impact of lifestyle changes and medication on long-term health [5, 6]. Diabetes Control and Complications Trial (DCCT) and 'The United Kingdom Prospective Diabetes Study' (UKPDS) demonstrated the utility of HbA1c in screening of diabetes and its associated complications. Specific targets have been set for HbA_1c for the management of DM [7, 8].

Studies including UKPDS and DCCT claimed that for every 1% reduction in HbA_1c value, there is a 37% reduction in micro-vascular complications especially incidence of diabetic retinopathy. It has been understood from a different study that sustained hyperglycemia is an important determinant of the long-term complications that have renewed interest in monitoring the control of diabetes [7, 9, 10].

In patients with type 1 diabetes mellitus (T1DM), HbA1c is the major limiting factor in attaining reasonable glycemic control [10]. In one of the previously published studies named The Diabetes Control and Complications Trial (DCCT), quadratic association was observed between HbA1c and the severe hypoglycemia which in brief demonstrates that when the HbA1c decreased the severity of hypoglycemia is increased [11, 12]. The results of this study were again attested by the EURODIAB IDDM complication study in which it was observed that 40.1% of patients having HbA1c of 36 mmol/mol (5.4%) were found affected by severe hypoglycemia compared to HbA1c of 24.3% patients with a limit of 62 mmol/mol (7.8%) [13]. On other hand, a contradictory recent study showed no significant association between HbA1c and hypoglycemia in children and adults [14–18]. Importantly, several other studies indicate that other factors, such as hypoglycemia awareness status and duration of diabetes, might be more important in identifying individuals prone to severe hypoglycemia [19–21].

In another study named as Action to Control Cardiovascular Risk in Diabetes (ACCORD), it was observed that episodes of severe hypoglycemia increase the risk for developing cardiovascular episodes and mortality in patients with type 2 diabetes mellitus having high concentrations of HbA1c concentrations. Until now, nonetheless, not many examinations have investigated whether shifting HbA1c values might represent various lengths of hypoglycemia in type 2 diabetic patients getting hypoglycemic medications that could cause hypoglycemia. In one of the previous studies, authors administered basal-bolus treatment as surveyed by concealed CGM and found that few study participants have a middle HbA1c worth of 52 mmol/mol (6.9%) (range, 6.3–8.6). Considering that both the scope of postprandial glucose increment and the chance to postprandial pinnacle glucose values were demonstrated to be most noteworthy after breakfast in these patients, reasoning is recommended for focusing on post-breakfast glucose increments for treatment in type 1 diabetic patients.

The objectives of glucose-bringing down treatment in type 2 diabetes are to diminish the gamble of diabetes confusions while limiting damages related with treatment and consequently increment both life span and well-being-related personal satisfaction. Concentrated glucose-bringing down systems unobtrusively decrease the gamble of substitutes for micro-vascular difficulties, yet the advantages for macro-vascular results are less clear [12, 22–25]. A new position explanation from the American Diabetes Affiliation (ADA) has called for individualized dynamic in diabetes that coordinates patient objectives and inclinations and considers the advantages and dangers related to treatment to set glycemic focuses for care [26]. The ADA and American Geriatrics Society have made comparative suggestions for more seasoned patients with diabetes [27]. In any case, information was missing on the best way to individualize glycemic targets. A few examinations of observational information have zeroed in on figuring out what concentrations of glycemic control boost benefits [28, 29]; however, less is realized about the dangers related to different degrees of glucose control. Hypoglycemia is the most widely recognized antagonistic impact of diabetes treatment and is related with ominous well-being results (higher gamble of dementia, falls, fall-related cracks, cardiovascular occasions, chronic weakness–related personal satisfaction, and expanded mortality). Accordingly, information on the connection between glucose control and chance of serious hypoglycemia is basic for coming to educated conclusions about type and power regarding treatment [30–37].

Study participants with having lower-side HbA1c were presented by high episodes of hypoglycemia. On contradictory, DCCT stated an inverse association between HbA1c and extreme episodes of hypoglycemia especially in participants with type 1 diabetes. Randomized controlled studies performed in preliminary settings demonstrated that in both type 1 and type 2 diabetes mellitus lower HbA1c is positively associated with frequency of hypoglycemia episodes. In of the pioneer ACCORD trial, it has been observed that increased hypoglycemia risk in type 2 diabetic participants with poorer glycemic control compared with subjects with more desirable HbA1c levels [38]. In this trial, both arms, (treatment and the control) showed poor glycemic control with the hypoglycemia events. Earlier observational examinations have yielded clashing outcomes; some have demonstrated expanded hazard of hypoglycemia at lower HbA1c concentrations [39], while others have shown positive associations between HbA1c and hypoglycemia, yet these earlier investigations were not really explicitly intended to test the relationship among HbA1c and hypoglycemia. In addition, most examinations depended on hypoglycemic occasions that came to clinical consideration (as determined from crisis division or medical clinic records) and in this manner might miss most of occasions that are treated beyond the clinical framework.

2. Structure of glycosylated hemoglobin

There are many different types of glycosylated hemoglobin. All the glycosylated hemoglobins have a carbohydrate moiety (glucose or a derivative) attached to one of the globin chains through glycation. Glycation is the nonenzymatic reaction in which the addition of glucose to amino groups of proteins takes place. HbA_1c is glycated hemoglobin in which glucose is bound specifically to the N-terminal valine of the hemoglobin β chain. HbA_1c constitutes the major portion of the glycated hemoglobin [40]. The heterogeneity of hemoglobin of human beings has been demonstrated for the first time by Allen et al. in 1958 using cation exchange chromatography. Similar results were obtained using electrophoresis by other scientists, which established the identity between Hb fractions separated by chromatography and by electrophoresis. Experiments showed that there was a major difference between the elution of minor Hb peaks and major HbA fraction. Minor Hb is known as 'fast hemoglobins' or HbA1, and major Hb were eventually called as HbAo [40]. These peaks were named based on their chromatographic elution order. After several experiments, it was highlighted

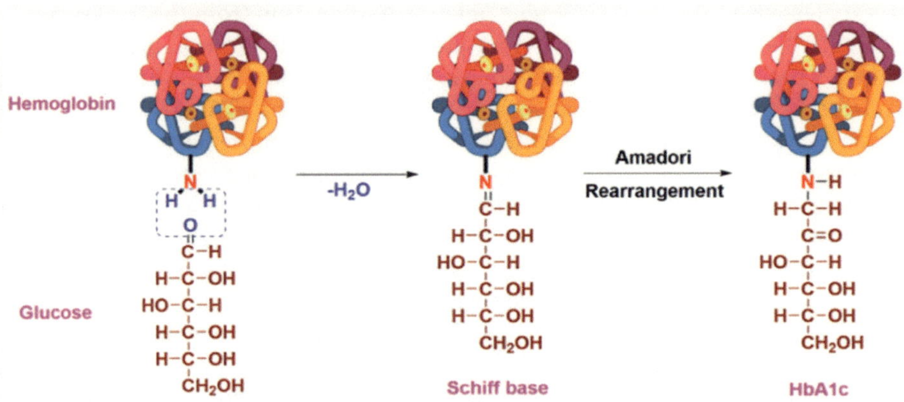

Figure 1.
Non-enzymatic glycosylation of Hb (adopted from Ref. [44] under the terms and conditions of the Creative Commons Attribution (CC BY) license (https://creativecommons.org/licenses/by/4.0/).

that these Hb fractions are formed by the combination of the different components to HbA leading to change in the physiological and biochemical properties of the molecule, which is also a basis for their separation. It was unequivocally discovered that glucose is the major compound responsible for the formation of HbA1c, also considered to be an Amadori product formed by the binding of glucose to the β -N-terminal valine residues of globin chains, rearranged into 1-deoxy-1-N-valyl-fructose and present in the ring form [41]. The bonding is irreversible so it cannot be dissociated. Similarly, HbA1a1 and HbA1a2 were characterized by the binding of fructose-1,6-bisphosphate and glucose6-phosphate to the β globin N-terminal extremities of hemoglobin, respectively. Other normal hemoglobin species like HbA 2 and HbF are also glycated like HbA; however, the glycation kinetics is different. Advanced glycation end products (AGEs) is formed by a continuous process of the anabolism of carbohydrates with proteins especially with long half-lives mainly by oxidative processes, which plays a major role in degenerative long-term complications of diabetes mellitus and other chronic diseases [5, 41–43]. **Figure 1** demonstrates the structural alterations in Hb during non-enzymatic glycosylation.

3. Techniques to measure glycosylated hemoglobin

HbA1c can be separated easily based on a difference in net charge, unlike other HbA fractions. For the measurement of HbA_1c, whole blood samples are collected in EDTA vials that can be stored at 4°C for a week or at −70°C or colder for a period of one year. Methods used for the measurement of HbA_1c are boronate affinity method, enzymatic method, affinity chromatography, high-performance liquid chromatography, isoelectric focusing radioimmunoassay, spectrophotometric assay, and electrophoresis/electroendosmosis.

3.1 Boronate affinity method

Boronate affinity chromatography is among the priority methods that is not influenced by the presence of other Hb variants [42, 43, 45]. In this method, m-amino phenylboronic acid reacts specifically with the cis-diol groups of glucose bound to Hb. This method measures total glycated GHB, including HbA_1c and Hb glycated at other sites [46].

3.2 Enzymatic method

It measures HbA1c by using an enzyme that specifically cleaves the N-terminal valine [5, 41–43].

3.3 Affinity chromatography

In this method, the diol moieties in glycosylated hemoglobins are absorbed selectively, allowing separation from unmodified hemoglobin. This technique is less sensitive to changes in temperature and pH, and the columns used in this method can be regenerated easily. It is mostly used to study diabetes in laboratory animals with heterogeneous hemoglobins that complicate assay by other methods [43].

3.4 High-performance liquid chromatography

Apart from being more costly and labor-intensive, HPLC method is a more sophisticated method that offers greater precision and allows the separation of the various components of HbA [42, 43, 45]. Ion-exchange HPLC separates Hb species based on charge differences between HbA1c and other hemoglobins.

3.5 Isoelectric focusing

Isoelectric focusing is valuable as a research method because of its high resonance. The main advantage of this method is that it can identify different variants and HbA_1c is readily separated from the intermediate Schiff base [42, 43, 45].

3.6 Radioimmunoassay

For measuring HbA_1c through radioimmunoassay, a specific antibody is required. The method has not yet been developed for general use. Most of the available immunoassays measure HbA_1c specifically by antibodies that recognize the structure of the N-terminal glycated amino acids of the Hb β chain.

3.7 Spectrophotometric assay

This method is based on phytic acid-binding to hemoglobin and its optical absorption properties as glycosylated hemoglobin does not bind phytic acid. The method requires a precision spectrophotometer with high resolution [42, 43, 45].

3.8 Electrophoresis/electroendosmosis

Conventional electrophoretic techniques have not proved suitable for the assay of Hb A as glycosylation of hemoglobin changes its isoelectric point by only 0–01 pH unit. Also, in the modern era, reading of the plates requires the careful setting of the scanning densitometer to the correct baseline [42, 43, 45].

There is a requirement of the reference range for each method. It may be possible that there may not even be a linear relationship between results obtained using different methods. The optimum incubation temperature, dilution, and length of time necessary is a topic of research these days.

4. Application in management of diabetes

The glycosylated hemoglobin is simple, objective, and representative of average blood glucose concentrations over several weeks and is considered a reliable yardstick of diabetic control. As the normal life span of red blood cells (RBCs) is 90–120 days, therefore HbA1c predicts the average glucose level of 90 days period. As per American Diabetes Association, for best management of diabetes patients, the target of HbA1c should be below 53 mmol/mol (7%); however, for diagnosis purpose, subjects with HbA1C level less than 39 mmol/mol (5.7%) are categorized as subjects with normal glucose tolerance, and between 39 mmol/mol (5.7) and less than 48 mmol/mol (6.5%) have been considered to be prediabetic, while A1C level of 48 mmol/mol (6.5%) or higher represents diabetes range [1]. It is independent of patient compliance and not affected by short-term fluctuation if steps are taken to remove aldimine [43, 45, 46]. Freedom from the dramatic short-term complications of diabetes (ketoacidosis and hypoglycemia) cannot be guaranteed as good diabetes control. Many patients will feel perfectly well even after having blood glucose concentrations in the mid or upper teens (mmol/l) for long periods [45–47]. Random blood glucose measurements, especially in insulin-treated patients, have considerable fluctuations even during a single day and can be quite misleading. The home urine testing is also unreliable in terms of diabetes control. There are very few patients motivated enough to present to the clinic with carefully recorded values of regular glucose testing. As the renal threshold is not constant, even reliably collected results may still be misleading. Although HbA1c is a useful parameter in terms of whether overall glucose control is good or bad, it neither specifies at what time of day blood glucose is high nor specifically indicates that any event of hypoglycemia has occurred [41]. At the same time, we cannot estimate the overall blood glucose control status through the blood glucose value taken at any specific time. Therefore, HbA_1c and regular home blood glucose monitoring should be looked upon together, each complementing the information provided by the other.

The main advantage of HbA_1c is that it is not affected or least affected by the blood fluctuating concentrations and other medical conditions. However, some factors affect the HbA1c concentrations. The life span of erythrocytes can affect the HbA_1c values. Other factors like anemia in patients with chronic kidney disease, hemolytic anemia, on erythropoietin use can also affect the HbA_1c concentrations. Iron deficiency can also correlate with false HbA_1c values. Pregnancy is also among the major contributing factors for false reading of HbA_1c [43].

5. Significance of HbA1c in hypoglycemia

It has been observed that hypoglycemia is primarily occurred due to overutilization of metabolic fuel glucose due to hyperinsulinism and significant reduction of blood sugar concentrations that directly affect the hemoglobin structure and thereby take part in chemical modifications of hemoglobin. This chemical

HbA_{1c} 'old'	HbA_{1c} 'new'	HbA_{1c} 'old'	HbA_{1c} 'new'
4.0	20	9.1	76
4.1	21	9.2	77
4.2	22	9.3	78
4.3	23	9.4	79
4.4	25	9.5	80
4.5	26	9.6	81
4.6	27	9.7	83
4.7	28	9.8	84
4.8	29	9.9	85
4.9	30	10.0	86
5.0	31	10.1	87
5.1	32	10.2	88
5.2	33	10.3	89
5.3	34	10.4	90
5.4	36	10.5	91
5.5	37	10.6	92
5.6	38	10.7	93
5.7	39	10.8	95
5.8	40	10.9	96
5.9	41	11.0	97
6.0	42	11.1	98
6.1	43	11.2	99
6.2	44	11.3	100
6.3	45	11.4	101
6.4	46	11.5	102
6.5	48	11.6	103
6.6	49	11.7	104
6.7	50	11.8	105
6.8	51	11.9	107
6.9	52	12.0	108
7.0	53	13.0	119
7.1	54	13.1	120
7.2	55	13.2	121
7.3	56	13.3	122
7.4	57	13.4	123
7.5	58	13.5	124
7.6	60	13.6	125
7.7	61	13.7	126
7.8	62	13.8	127
7.9	63	13.9	128

HbA_{1c} 'old'	HbA_{1c} 'new'	HbA_{1c} 'old'	HbA_{1c} 'new'
8.0	64	14.0	130
8.1	65	14.1	131
8.2	66	14.2	132
8.3	67	14.3	133
8.4	68	14.4	134
8.5	69	14.5	135
8.6	70	14.6	136
8.7	72	14.7	137
8.8	73	14.8	138
8.9	74	14.9	139
9.0	75		

Table 1.
Glycated hemoglobin conversion table: Older DCCT-aligned (%) and newer IFCC-standardized (mmol/Mol) concentrations (adopted from Ref [48]).

modification pathway is contributed in two ways (1) reduced concentrations of blood glucose cause proportional decreases in concentrations of glycosylated hemoglobin and (2) simultaneous significant perturbations of a part of hemoglobin take place. Therefore, in the episodes of hypoglycemia due to varying reasons causes lowering concentrations of glycosylated hemoglobin compared to the hyperglycemia and normoglycemia. HbA1c in case of hypoglycemia reflects the mean blood glucose concentrations as in hyperglycemia. Further studies are needed in this direction to establish a strong relationship between hypoglycemia and glycated hemoglobin that can be used in diagnosis and characterization of hypoglycemia and also its management. In one of the previously published studies, it was found that the amounts of HbA, in hypoglycemia samples, were found to be higher than expected from the correlation that is known to exist between the amount of sugar bound to the total Hb and the 'amount of HbA' in normal and diabetic samples [29]. This may be of practical interest in biomedicine, particularly when HbA, measurements are used for glucose level estimates in diabetic patients with frequent episodes of hypoglycemia (**Table 1**) [49–52].

6. Conclusion

Glycosylated hemoglobin currently is a gold standard method for management and diagnosis of diabetes mellitus worldwide. While some obstacles remain in the analysis of HbA_1c, it has come a long way over the past few decades. With the development of the international harmonization, HbA_1c assessment got recognition in the guidelines and is currently recommended as a test for diagnosis, assessment, and management of diabetes mellitus. Moreover, with some cofounding interfering factors, still, HbA_1c is one of the best choices for clinicians and physicians. Several sophisticated research methods for quantification of HbA1c are available that are very efficient and effective in measuring the concentrations of HbA_1c with higher specificity and sensitivity.

Acknowledgements

The authors AR and GBJ want to thank the Brain Pool Program funded by the Ministry of Science and ICT through the National Research Foundation of Korea (Grant Number—KRF 2022H1D3A2A01096346) for supporting this research.

Conflict of interest

The authors declare no conflict of interest.

Author details

Brijesh Kumar Mishra[1†], Alok Raghav[2*†], Goo-Bo Jeong[2], Mukesh Jain[1], Pinky Shukla[1] and Swati Sharma[3]

1 Department of Endocrinology, UCMS and GTB Hospital, Delhi, India

2 Department of Anatomy and Cell Biology, Lee Gill Ya Cancer and Diabetes Institute, Gachon University, Incheon, South Korea

3 Homi Bhabha Cancer Hospital, Varanasi, India

*Address all correspondence to: alokalig@gmail.com

† Equal contribution.

References

[1] Care D, Suppl SS. Classification and diagnosis of diabetes: Standards of medical care in Diabetesd 2018. Diabetes Care. 2018;**41**(January):S13-S27. DOI: 10.2337/dc18-S002

[2] Wild S, Roglic G, Green A, Sicree R, King H. Global prevalence of diabetes: Estimates for the year 2000 and projections for 2030. Diabetes Care. 2004;**27**(5):1047-1053. DOI: 10.2337/diacare.27.5.1047

[3] Gebel E. The start of something good: The discovery of HbA1c and the American Diabetes Association Samuel Rahbar outstanding discovery award. Diabetes Care. 2012;**35**(12):2429-2431. DOI: 10.2337/dc12-1763

[4] John WG, Mosca A, Weykamp C, Goodall I. HbA1c standardisation: history, science and politics. Clinical Biochemist Reviews. Nov 2007;**28**(4):163-168

[5] Gillery P. A history of HbA 1c through clinical chemistry and laboratory medicine. Clinical Chemistry and Laboratory Medicine. 2013;**51**(1):65-74. DOI: 10.1515/cclm-2012-0548

[6] Lundholm MD, Emanuele MA, Ashraf A, Nadeem S. Applications and pitfalls of hemoglobin A1C and alternative methods of glycemic monitoring. Journal of Diabetes and Its Complications. Aug 2020;**34**(8):107585

[7] King P, Peacock I, Donnelly R. The UK prospective diabetes study (UKPDS): Clinical and therapeutic implications for type 2 diabetes. British Journal of Clinical Pharmacology. Nov 1999;**48**(5):643-648

[8] Lautsch D, Boggs R, Wang T, Gonzalez C, Milligan G, Rajpathak S, et al. Individualized HbA_{1c} goals, and patient awareness and attainment of goals in type 2 diabetes mellitus: A real-world multinational survey. Advances in Therapy. 2022;**39**(2):1016-1032. DOI: 10.1007/s12325-021-01985-3

[9] Kojić Damjanov S, Đerić M, Eremić KN. Glycated hemoglobin A1c as a modern biochemical marker of glucose regulation. Medicinski Pregled. 2014;**67**(9-10):339-344. DOI: 10.2298/MPNS1410339K

[10] Ghazanfari Z, Haghdoost AA, Alizadeh SM, Atapour J, Zolala F. A Comparison of HbA1c and Fasting Blood Sugar Tests in General Population. International Journal of Preventive Medicine. 2010 Summer;**1**(3):187-194

[11] Cryer PE. Hypoglycaemia: The limiting factor in the glycaemic management of type I and type II diabetes. Diabetologia. 2002;**45**:937-948

[12] The Diabetes Control and Complications Trial Research Group. The effect of intensive treatment of diabetes on the development and progression of long-term complications in insulin-dependent diabetes mellitus. The New England Journal of Medicine. 1993;**329**:977-986

[13] The Diabetes Control and Complications Trial Research Group. Hypoglycemia in the diabetes control and complications trial. Diabetes. 1997;**46**:271-286

[14] EUROBIAB IDDM Complications Study Group. Microvascular and acute complications in IDDM patients: The EURODIAB IDDM complications study. Diabetologia. 1994;**37**:278-285

[15] Miller KM, Foster NC, Beck RW, Bergenstal RM, DuBose SN, DiMeglio LA, et al. Current state of type 1 diabetes treatment in the U.S.: Updated data from the T1D exchange clinic registry. Diabetes Care. 2015;**38**:971-978

[16] Weinstock RS, Xing D, Maahs DM, Michels A, Rickels MR, Peters AL, et al. Severe hypoglycemia and diabetic ketoacidosis in adults with type 1 diabetes: Results from the T1D exchange clinic registry. The Journal of Clinical Endocrinology and Metabolism. 2013;**98**:3411-3419

[17] Simmons JH, Chen V, Miller KM, McGill JB, Bergenstal RM, Goland RS, et al. Differences in the management of type 1 diabetes among adults under excellent control compared with those under poor control in the T1D exchange clinic registry. Diabetes Care. 2013;**36**:3573-3577. Available from: https://www.ncbi.nlm.nih.gov/pubmed/?term=PLoS+Med+11%2C+2014%2C+e1001742

[18] Campbell MS, Schatz DA, Chen V, Wong JC, Steck A, Tamborlane WV, et al. A contrast between children and adolescents with excellent and poor control: The T1D exchange clinic registry experience. Pediatric Diabetes. 2014;**15**:110-117

[19] Gold AE, MacLeod KM, Frier BM. Frequency of severe hypoglycemia in patients with type I diabetes with impaired awareness of hypoglycemia. Diabetes Care. 1994;**17**:697-703

[20] Pedersen-Bjergaard U, Pramming S, Heller SR, Wallace TM, Rasmussen AK, Jorgensen HV, et al. Severe hypoglycaemia in 1076 adult patients with type 1 diabetes: Influence of risk markers and selection. Diabetes/Metabolism Research and Reviews. 2004;**20**:479-486

[21] UK Hypoglycaemia Study Group. Risk of hypoglycaemia in types 1 and 2 diabetes: Effects of treatment modalities and their duration. Diabetologia. 2007;**50**:1140-1147

[22] van Beers CA, DeVries JH, Kleijer SJ, Smits MM, Geelhoed-Duijvestijn PH, Kramer MH, et al. Continuous glucose monitoring for patients with type 1 diabetes and impaired awareness of hypoglycaemia (IN CONTROL): A randomised, open-label, crossover trial. The Lancet Diabetes and Endocrinology. 2016;**4**:893-902

[23] Duckworth W, Abraira C, Moritz T, Reda D, Emanuele N, Reaven PD, et al. Glucose control and vascular complications in veterans with type 2 diabetes. The New England Journal of Medicine. 2009;**360**(2):129-139

[24] Action to Control Cardiovascular Risk in Diabetes Study Group, Gerstein HC, Miller ME, Byington RP, Goff DC Jr, Bigger JT, et al. Effects of intensive glucose lowering in type 2 diabetes. The New England Journal of Medicine. 2008;**358**(24):2545-2559

[25] ADVANCE Collaborative Group, Patel A, MacMahon S, Chalmers J, Neal B, Billot L, et al. Intensive blood glucose control and vascular outcomes in patients with type 2 diabetes. The New England Journal of Medicine. 2008;**358**(24):2560-2572

[26] Intensive blood-glucose control with sulphonylureas or insulin compared with conventional treatment and risk of complications in patients with type 2 diabetes (UKPDS 33). UK Prospective Diabetes Study (UKPDS) Group. Lancet. 1998;**352**(9131):837-853. Erratum in: Lancet 1999 Aug 14;354(9178):602

[27] Inzucchi SE, Bergenstal RM, Buse JB, Diamant M, Ferrannini E, Nauck M,

et al. Management of hyperglycemia in type 2 diabetes: A patient-centered approach: Position statement of the American Diabetes Association (ADA) and the European Association for the Study of diabetes (EASD). Diabetes Care. 2012;**35**(6):1364-1379

[28] Kirkman MS, Briscoe VJ, Clark N, Florez H, Haas LB, Halter JB, et al. Diabetes in older adults. Diabetes Care. 2012;**35**(12):2650-2664

[29] Greenfield S, Billimek J, Pellegrini F, Franciosi M, De Berardis G, Nicolucci A, et al. Comorbidity affects the relationship between glycemic control and cardiovascular outcomes in diabetes: A cohort study. Annals of Internal Medicine. 2009;**151**(12):854-860

[30] Huang ES, Liu JY, Moffet HH, John PM, Karter AJ. Glycemic control, complications, and death in older diabetic patients: The diabetes and aging study. Diabetes Care. 2011 Jun;**34**(6):1329-1336

[31] Whitmer RA, Karter AJ, Yaffe K, Quesenberry CP Jr, Selby JV. Hypoglycemic episodes and risk of dementia in older patients with type 2 diabetes mellitus. Journal of the American Medical Association. 2009;**301**(15):1565-1572

[32] Schwartz AV, Vittinghoff E, Sellmeyer DE, Feingold KR, de Rekeneire N, Strotmeyer ES, et al. Diabetes-related complications, glycemic control, and falls in older adults. Diabetes Care. 2008;**31**(3):391-396. DOI: 10.2337/dc07-1152. Epub 2007 Dec 4. Erratum in: Diabetes Care. 2008 May;31(5):1089

[33] Johnston SS, Conner C, Aagren M, Ruiz K, Bouchard J. Association between hypoglycaemic events and fall-related fractures in Medicare-covered patients with type 2 diabetes. Diabetes, Obesity & Metabolism. 2012;**14**(7):634-643

[34] Johnston SS, Conner C, Aagren M, Smith DM, Bouchard J, Brett J. Evidence linking hypoglycemic events to an increased risk of acute cardiovascular events in patients with type 2 diabetes. Diabetes Care. 2011;**34**(5):1164-1170

[35] Desouza C, Salazar H, Cheong B, Murgo J, Fonseca V. Association of hypoglycemia and cardiac ischemia: A study based on continuous monitoring. Diabetes Care. 2003;**26**(5):1485-1489

[36] Green AJ, Fox KM, Grandy S, SHIELD Study Group. Self-reported hypoglycemia and impact on quality of life and depression among adults with type 2 diabetes mellitus. Diabetes Research and Clinical Practice. 2012;**96**(3):313-318

[37] Laiteerapong N, Karter AJ, Liu JY, Moffet HH, Sudore R, Schillinger D, et al. Correlates of quality of life in older adults with diabetes: The diabetes & aging study. Diabetes Care. 2011;**34**(8):1749-1753

[38] McCoy RG, Van Houten HK, Ziegenfuss JY, Shah ND, Wermers RA, Smith SA. Increased mortality of patients with diabetes reporting severe hypoglycemia. Diabetes Care. 2012;**35**(9):1897-1901

[39] Miller ME, Bonds DE, Gerstein HC, Seaquist ER, Bergenstal RM, Calles-Escandon J, et al. The effects of baseline characteristics, glycaemia treatment approach, and glycated haemoglobin concentration on the risk of severe hypoglycaemia: Post hoc epidemiological analysis of the ACCORD study. BMJ. 2010;**8**(340):b5444

[40] Allen DW, Schroeder WA, Balog J. Observations on the chromatographic

heterogeneity of normal adult and fetal human hemoglobin: a study of the effects of crystallization and chromatography on the heterogeneity and isoleucine content. Journal of the American Chemical Society. 1958;**80**:1628-1634

[41] Kosmachevskaya OV, Novikova NN, Topunov AF. Carbonyl stress in red blood cells and hemoglobin. Antioxidants. 2021;**10**(2):1-23. DOI: 10.3390/antiox10020253 842 Structure and Nomenclature Ofhemoglobin Variants Name

[42] Sacks DB. Measurement of hemoglobin A1c: A new twist on the path to harmony. Diabetes Care. 2012;**35**(12):2674-2680. DOI: 10.2337/dc12-1348

[43] Peacock I. Glycosylated hemoglobin: Measurement and clinical use. Journal of Clinical Pathology. 1984;**37**(8):841-851. DOI: 10.1136/jcp.37.8.841

[44] Mandali PK, Prabakaran A, Annadurai K, Krishnan UM. Trends in quantification of HbA1c using electrochemical and point-of-Care analyzers. Sensors. 1901;**2023**:23. DOI: 10.3390/s23041901

[45] Little RR, Roberts WL. A review of variant Hemoglobins interfering with hemoglobin A1c measurement. Available from: www.journalofdst.org

[46] Leow MKS. Glycated hemoglobin (HbA1c): Clinical applications of a mathematical concept. Acta Informatica Medica. 2016;**24**(4):233-238. DOI: 10.5455/aim.2016.24.233-238

[47] Sudhakar Nayak S, Pattabirarnan TN. A new calorimetric method for the estimation of glycosylated hemoglobin. Clinica Chimica Acta. 1981;**109**:267-274

[48] Riemsma R, Corro Ramos I, Birnie R, Büyükkaramikli N, Armstrong N, Ryder S et al. Integrated sensor-augmented pump therapy systems [the MiniMed® Paradigm™ Veo system and the Vibe™ and G4® PLATINUM CGM (continuous glucose monitoring) system] for managing blood glucose levels in type 1 diabetes: a systematic review and economic evaluation. Health Technol Assess. Feb 2016;**20**(17):v-xxxi, 1-251

[49] Hanas R. John G; international HBA1c consensus committee. 2010 consensus statement on the worldwide standardization of the hemoglobin A1C measurement. Diabetes Care. 2010;**33**(8):1903-1904. DOI: 10.2337/dc10-0953

[50] Frier BM, Ratzki-Leewing A, Harris SB. Reporting of hypoglycaemia in clinical trials of basal insulins: A need for consensus. Diabetes, Obesity & Metabolism. 2019;**21**(7):1529-1542. DOI: 10.1111/dom.13732. Epub 2019 Apr 29

[51] Perlman JE, Gooley TA, McNulty B, Meyers J, Hirsch IB. HbA1c and glucose management indicator discordance: A real-world analysis. Diabetes Technology & Therapeutics. 2021;**23**(4):253-258. DOI: 10.1089/dia.2020.0501

[52] Šoupal J, Petruželková L, Grunberger G, Hásková A, Flekač M, Matoulek M, et al. Glycemic outcomes in adults with T1D are impacted more by continuous glucose monitoring than by insulin delivery method: 3 years of follow-up from the COMISAIR study. Diabetes Care. 2020;**43**(1):37-43. DOI: 10.2337/dc19-0888

Chapter 6

Perspective Chapter: Crosstalk between Bone Metabolism and Insulin Resistance

Venera Berisha-Muharremi

Abstract

Bone has traditionally been considered a passive organ, serving only as a scaffold for other organs and the entire body. However, over the past few years, an increasing number of studies have highlighted its function as an endocrine organ regulating energy and adipose tissue metabolism by producing undercarboxylated osteocalcin (ucOC). In mice, ucOC administration through different routes has been explored for its potential as a therapeutic or preventive method for reducing adipocyte size and normalising glucose homeostasis. The discovery of these endocrine properties of ucOC in rodent models for obesity prevention and treatment necessitates evaluating the association of ucOC with insulin resistance and obesity-related parameters in humans. This study aimed to investigate the association between total osteocalcin and ucOC, which is proposed as the active form in rodent models, with glucose metabolism markers, insulin resistance, and obesity-related parameters (i.e. Haemoglobin A1c, fasting glucose, and insulin resistance evaluated by homeostasis model assessment) in individuals who are overweight or obese. This study concluded the possible correlation of ucOC, with insulin resistance and highlights that waist/hip ratio can be a predictor of ucOC.

Keywords: osteocalcin, undercarboxylated osteocalcin, bone metabolism, insulin resistance, obesity

1. Introduction

The number of people suffering from metabolic syndrome (MetSy) is increasing globally. MetSy is a group of risk factors for various conditions, including insulin resistance, hypertension, high triglyceride levels, low high-density lipoprotein levels, and abdominal obesity, where the key problem seems to be insulin resistance. These factors put individuals at a higher risk of developing cardiovascular disease and type 2 diabetes (T2D) [1].

Recent studies have suggested the existence of a close relationship between bone metabolism and the metabolism of energy, glycaemia, and insulin, mediated by osteocalcin (OC) [2, 3]. Endocrinologists have traditionally considered bone an organ, where the actions of only classic hormones (such as steroids, parathyroid hormone, and calcitonin) were known. Bones were considered merely a part of the skeleton, a supportive system.

However, results from research in the past few decades have demonstrated that bone mass is also regulated by fat through leptin, which acts upon the brain, and downstream through the hypothalamic relay and sympathetic nervous system [4–7]. Based on these findings, from an endocrine perspective, it can be speculated that there is a feedback mechanism. Indeed, research and experiments involving rodent models suggest a new possible role for bone by producing OC, which acts as a hormone that influences insulin production and sensitivity, glucose utilisation, and energy expenditure [6–8]. Reviews of these findings have been published [6–11].

OC (also called bone γ-carboxyglutamic acid protein) is a bone protein secreted by osteoblasts consisting of 46–50 residues (**Figure 1**) [6, 7, 12] that undergoes posttranslational modification by vitamin K dependent γ-carboxylation of three glutamic acid residues [6, 7, 13]. Undercarboxylated osteocalcin (ucOC), which is the OC form with a lower binding affinity to bone, has fewer than three carboxylated residues [5–7]. In human serum, both forms can be found and measured. OC, until recently, was used only as a useful marker of bone formation. It is expressed by mature osteoblasts, binds strongly to hydroxyapatite, is stored in the bone matrix, and is released into the circulation [5–7].

Mutant mice without osteocalcin ($OC^{-/-}$ mice) show no remarkable bone phenotype but appear hyperglycaemic and have increased visceral fat [6, 7, 14]. On the other hand, mutant mice with deletion of the *Esp* gene ($Esp^{-/-}$ mice), a gene encoding a receptor-like protein (osteotesticular protein tyrosine phosphatase [OST-PTP]), resulting in a phenotype opposite that of $OC^{-/-}$ mice. $Esp^{-/-}$ mice present with increased pancreatic islet size, β-cell number, and circulating insulin levels; increased insulin sensitivity despite hypoglycaemia; decreased visceral fat mass; increased expression of insulin target genes in the liver and muscle; increased energy expenditure; and unaffected food intake [2, 6, 7].

In ex vivo experiments, OC stimulates insulin expression in β cells and adiponectin, an adipokine whose overexpression enhances insulin sensitivity [6, 7, 15]. Insulin production and insulin sensitivity have been indicated to be enhanced by either OC addition or OC overproduction by osteoblasts. *In vivo* treatment of normal mice with non-γ-carboxylated OC generated by bacterial expression has resulted in increased pancreatic β-cell numbers, insulin secretion, energy expenditure, and insulin sensitivity, so it has the opposite effect on metabolism as that in $OC^{-/-}$ mice [6, 7, 16]. Hence, $Esp^{-/-}$ mice are also protected from diabetes, similar to treated mice with non-γ-carboxylated OC; alternately, bone-specific overexpression of OST-PTP results in a phenotype identical to that of $OC^{-/-}$ mice. Therefore, the hypothesis has been made that OST-PTP is responsible for inactivating OC through γ-carboxylation [3, 6, 7].

It can be summarised that OC can act and be considered a hormone. However, its regulation is not yet fully understood, and receptor-like proteins, such as OST-PTP,

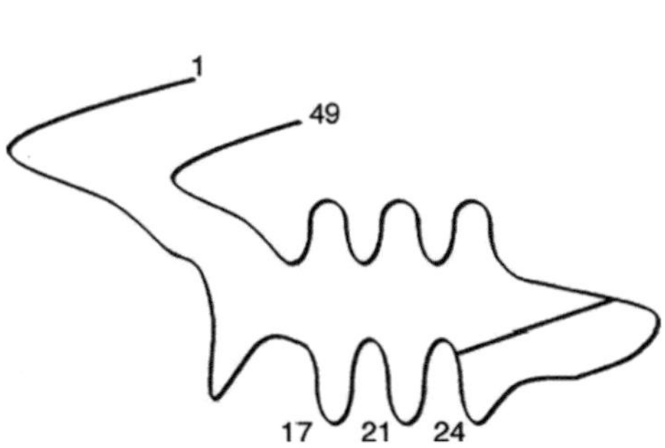

Figure 1.
Osteocalcin structure [6–8]. Three glutamic acid residues are present at positions 17, 21, and 24, and a disulphide bridge is present between residues 23 and 29.

may be involved in its signalling pathways, which are still unclear [6, 7]. The initial, definitive information about the role of OC, as a circulating hormone and especially its undercarboxylated fraction, in energy metabolism and particularly in the regulation of insulin secretion came from studies in mouse models where the experimental production of OC was either deactivated or increased [6, 7].

A similar OST-PTP as in mice has not been identified in humans. However, the OC level in human blood appears to be significantly lower in individuals with diabetes than in nondiabetic controls, and the level is inversely related to adiposity and blood glucose levels [6, 7, 17, 18]. Even in postmenopausal women, the OC level was significantly lower in subjects with T2D than in nondiabetic controls [19]. In a study that evaluated the effects of a hypocaloric diet and exercise, OC levels were positively associated with insulin sensitivity and negatively associated with triglyceride levels in a fasting state [20]. Serum OC level has been demonstrated to be associated with glucose metabolism and other atherosclerosis parameters in patients with T2D [21, 22]. Even in gestational diabetes, a higher OC level is observed compared to pregnancies with normal glucose levels [23]. In individuals with poorly controlled diabetes, only after 1 month of treatment and good glycaemic control was an increase in OC levels observed, while serum adiponectin did not show a difference before and after glycaemic control. However, the baseline level of adiponectin appears to predict the beneficial bone response [24]. Overall, in most studies, it can be concluded that the OC level increases in individuals with T2D after glycaemic control improvement [6, 7, 25–27].

Most publications on OC in humans were designed to study the effect of diabetes on bone remodelling and then, after the discovery of the endocrine effect, to retrospectively analyse the OC level of patients with diabetes [20, 21]. They were not initially designed to assess the effect of OC on insulin resistance or energy metabolism. Therefore, the exact role of OC in regulating insulin resistance cannot be conclusively determined yet and remains to be clarified.

Moreover, most previous clinical studies that have investigated the possible metabolic effects of OC did not differentiate total osteocalcin (TOC) from ucOC, which in rodents has been indicated to be the active form with metabolic effects. Experimental data has concluded that ucOC is involved in metabolism [3, 11]. Additionally, recent data from healthy children suggest a similar state in humans [28]. Studies in humans have indicated that improved glycaemic control increases the TOC level, but this does not necessarily mean that the same effect occurs for ucOC. Additional studies on the ucOC level are needed to clarify the effects of glycaemic control and insulin resistance improvement on this suggested hormone and vice versa.

TOC has been found to correlate with a decrease in insulin resistance and stimulate the production of insulin from the pancreas [12, 29]. Serum OC levels correlate with body mass index (BMI), C-reactive protein, insulin, and waist circumference [30]. OC levels have shown a significant negative correlation with insulin resistance (homeostasis model assessment for insulin resistance [HOMA-IR]) and waist/hip ratio [31]. Thus, serum OC levels in MetSy and insulin resistance could potentially be a new area to explore therapeutically. However, its role in clinical practice, especially the influence of the undercarboxylated form of this hormone on insulin sensitivity and vice versa, needs to be established.

This study, for the first time, aimed to investigate the relationship between not only TOC but also its supposed active fraction, ucOC, and insulin resistance as a companion occurrence of overweight and obesity in individuals without any medical treatment affecting their OC levels [32]. Furthermore, the study aimed to determine the correlation of both forms of OC with insulin resistance markers, glucose metabolism, and other obesity-related parameters in overweight and obese individuals [32].

2. Methodology

In a cross-sectional study, 123 consecutive persons, female ($n = 82$) and male ($n = 41$), with overweight and obesity (WHO criteria) [33] and aged 19–79 years were evaluated. The exclusion criteria were as follows: any pharmacologic treatments (not to interfere with study results), current or former smoking, pregnancy, and lactation, a history of type 1 diabetes mellitus, renal disease or renal failure, severe liver disease, HIV infection, known haematological diseases, eating disorders, or any psychiatric illness, functional thyroid disease, a history of bariatric surgery, malignancy, and metabolic bone disease.

Patient data were collected at Endomedica Polyclinic, Prishtina, Kosovo, between February 2022 and February 2023. The study was conducted in accordance with the Declaration of Helsinki and approved by the Committee of Ethics of the Faculty of Medicine, University of Prishtina, Kosovo (project identification code: 2679).

2.1 Clinical data: patient history

The data collected included answers to questions about the duration of overweight and obesity, family history, drug treatment, smoking, physical activity, and signs of other diseases or obesity complications. A physical examination was performed for each patient, including blood pressure measurements and measurements of weight, height, waist circumference, and hip circumference. Waist/hip ratio and BMI (weight [kg] divided by height^2 [m]) were calculated.

2.2 Analytical procedure: biochemical measurements

Blood was taken after a sober period at night. Commercial kits were used for biochemical parameters, and standard methods were recommended for routine biochemical tests. Fasting glucose, fasting insulin, Haemoglobin A1c (HbA1c), TOC, and ucOC levels were measured. Insulin resistance was assessed at the basal state—estimated by the homeostasis model assessment (HOMA) for insulin resistance (HOMA-IR), estimated steady state of β-cell function (HOMA%B), and insulin sensitivity (HOMA%S) [34] and calculated, using a downloaded calculator, from fasting blood glucose and fasting insulin level [35].

2.3 Statistical analyses

Median and interquartile range as variable summary parameters are used. A comparison between groups was made with the independent samples using the Mann-Whitney U test. The correlation between variables was tested with the Spearman correlation test, and linear regression tests were used to analyse the dependent variables: TOC and ucOC.

3. Results

The median age of the participants was 38 years (interquartile range: 30–45 years), and as shown in **Table 1**, no statistically significant difference was found between men and women ($p > .05$). Men were found to have higher levels of BMI, waist/hip ratio, HbA1c, Fasting blood glucose (FBG), insulin, β-cell function (HOMA%B), and insulin resistance (HOMA-IR) compared to women ($p < .05$; **Table 2**). However,

	Total N = 123			F n = 82			M n = 41			p
	Median	IQR		Median	IQR		Median	IQR		
Age (years)	38.00	30.00	45.00	38.00	29.00	49.25	36.00	30.50	43.50	.232
BMI (kg/m^2)	33.60	29.40	38.00	31.85	28.68	36.38	36.50	32.65	41.45	.001
Waist/hip ratio	1.00	0.90	1.10	0.90	0.90	1.00	1.10	1.10	1.30	<.0001
HbA1c (%)	5.40	5.06	6.09	5.20	4.90	6.00	5.80	5.21	6.25	.008
FBG (mmol/L)	5.40	5.00	5.90	5.30	4.92	5.83	5.72	5.20	6.10	.012
Insulin (μIU/L)	14.90	8.20	27.20	11.60	6.28	19.43	23.90	14.83	48.95	<.0001
HOMA%B	122.30	84.60	181.30	108.95	79.70	153.45	160.40	101.60	239.60	<.0001
HOMA%S	50.10	27.50	92.50	67.00	39.33	123.35	33.40	16.40	51.20	<.0001
HOMA-IR	2.00	1.08	3.60	1.52	0.80	2.53	2.99	1.95	6.10	<.0001
TOC (μg/L)	15.00	11.85	22.51	18.05	12.50	29.80	13.20	9.89	16.85	.001
ucOC (ng/mL)	1.12	0.65	1.60	1.44	0.98	2.09	0.58	0.36	1.02	<.0001

Table 1.
Comparison of measured parameters for both male and female patients. BMI—body mass index; HbA1c—Haemoglobin A1c; FBG—fasting blood glucose; HOMA%S—insulin sensitivity; HOMA%B—estimated steady state of β-cell function; HOMA-IR—insulin resistance.

		Age	BMI	Waist/hip ratio	HbA1c	FBG	Insulin	β-cell function	HOMA%S	HOMA-IR	TOC	ucOC
Age	r	1.000	.181	.090	.077	.245	.246	.110	−.268	.266	−.210	−.121
	p		.044	.320	.399	.006	.006	.228	.003	.003	.018	.180
BMI	r		1.000	.432	.499	.343	.559	.397	−.558	.557	−.356	−.458
	p			.000	.000	.000	.000	.000	.000	.000	.000	.000
Waist/hip ratio	r			1.000	.247	.333	.600	.424	−.595	.594	−.580	−.803
	p				.006	.000	.000	.000	.000	.000	.000	.000
HbA1c	r				1.000	.443	.385	.053	−.419	.417	−.222	−.235
	p					.000	.000	.558	.000	.000	.014	.009
FBG	r					1.000	.368	−.174	−.428	.425	−.206	−.248
	p						.000	.054	.000	.000	.022	.006
Insulin	r						1.000	.777	−.993	.994	−.600	−.762
	p							.000	.000	.000	.000	.000
HOMA%B	r							1.000	−.719	.721	−.440	−.610
	p								.000	.000	.000	.000
HOMA%S	r								1.000	−1.000	.603	.751
	p									.000	.000	.000
HOMA-IR	r									1.000	−.602	−.751
	p										.000	.000
TOC	r										1.000	.716
	p											.00
ucOC	r											1.000
	p											

Table 2.
Correlations of measured parameters. BMI—body mass index; HbA1c—Haemoglobin A1c; FBG—fasting blood glucose; HOMA%S—insulin sensitivity; HOMA%B—estimated steady state of β-cell function; HOMA-IR—insulin resistance; TOC—total osteocalcin; ucUC—undercarboxylated osteocalcin.

women had higher levels of HOMA%S, TOC, and ucOC compared to men ($p < .05$). About 32% of the men and 19% of the women in the study sample were in the obese class 3 category (**Figure 2**). Approximately 13% of the women and 15% of the men included in the study had hypertension (**Figure 3**). In addition, 8% of women and 12% of men had T2D (**Figure 4**).

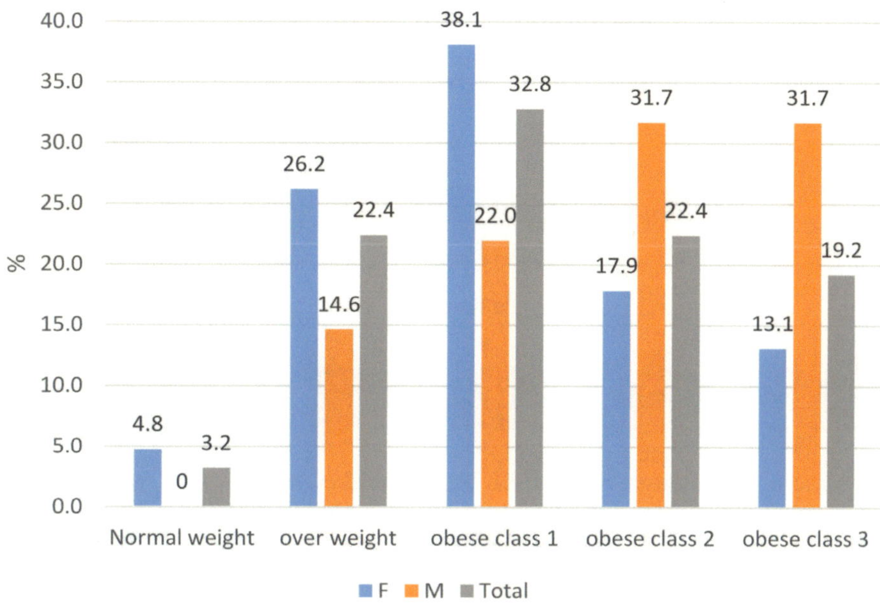

Figure 2.
Distribution based on body mass index.

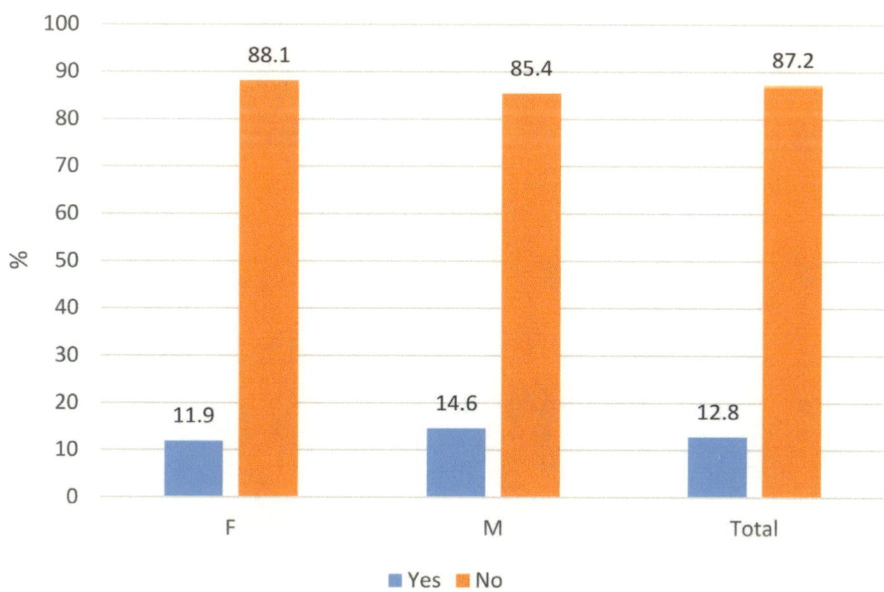

Figure 3.
The prevalence of hypertension among the study participants.

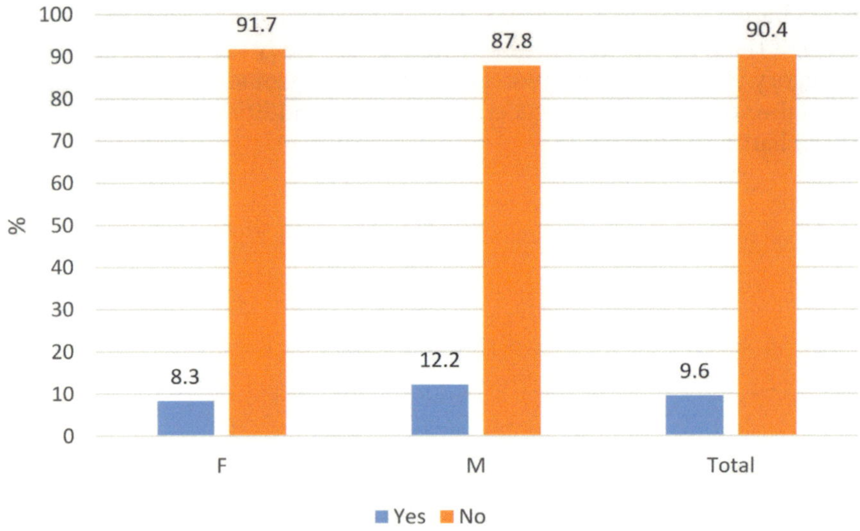

Figure 4.
The prevalence of diabetes among the study participants.

We found a low negative correlation of TOC with age, BMI, FBG, and HbA1c and a medium negative correlation with waist/hip ratio, insulin, β-cell function, and insulin resistance ($p < .05$). Furthermore, there was a medium correlation of TOC with HOMA%S ($p < .05$).

We found a low negative correlation of ucOC with FBG and HbA1c and a medium negative correlation with BMI and HOMA%B. However, ucOC was negatively correlated with insulin (**Figure 5**), and we found a very strong negative correlation between ucOC

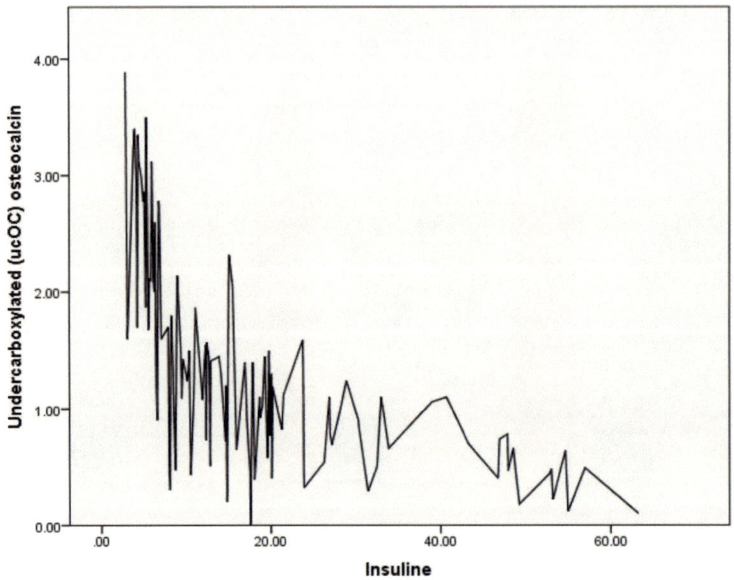

Figure 5.
Negative correlation between undercarboxylated osteocalcin and insulin.

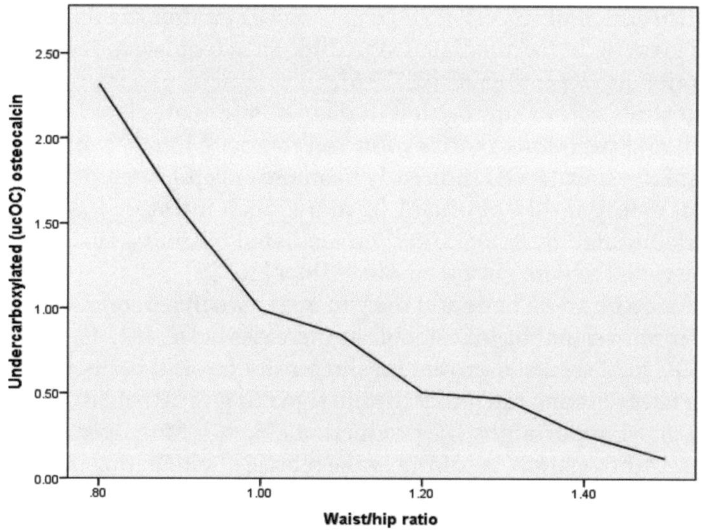

Figure 6.
Strong negative correlation between undercarboxylated osteocalcin and waist/hip ratio.

	Total osteocalcin		Undercarboxylated osteocalcin	
	B (95% CI)	P	B (95% CI)	P
Age	−0.127 (−0.245 to −0.010)	.034	—	—
Waist/hip ratio	−21.254 (−29.654 to −12.855)	<.0001	−2.506 (−3.137 to −1.875)	<.0001
HOMA%S	0.069 (0.040–0.097)	<.0001	0.013 (0.004–0.022)	.006
Insulin	—	—	0.012 (0.10–0.015)	<.0001

Table 3.
Correlation of total osteocalcin (TOC) and undercarboxylated osteocalcin (ucOC) with age, waist/hip ratio, homeostasis model assessment for insulin sensitivity (HOMA%S) value, and insulin level.

and waist/hip ratio (**Figure 6**). In addition, there was a strong positive correlation between ucOC and HOMA%S ($p < .05$). Multiple linear regression analyses indicated that age, waist/hip ratio, and HOMA%S are significant predicting factors for TOC, and according to the results, waist/hip ratio can predict ucOC (**Table 3**).

4. Discussion

The knowledge that ucOC secreted from bone regulates glucose metabolism dates back to studies by the Karsenty group—which generated, for the first time, rodent models without OC and revealed that these mutant OC-null mice accumulated abnormal amounts of visceral fat and exhibited severe glucose metabolism impairments [6, 7, 13, 36]. Because ucOC is an osteoblast-produced protein that enters the general circulation during bone remodelling [12, 36], it was speculated that ucOC is a hormone.

Studies with genetically modified rodent models have revealed that β cells in the pancreas are one of the major targets of ucOC as a hormone [36]. In OC $^{-/-}$ mice, all the effects are reduced, including insulin secretion into the circulation; islet number; β-cell area, mass, and proliferation; and pancreatic insulin content [6, 7, 36].

In contrast, mice deficient in OST-PTP (Esp $^{-/-}$ mice) exhibit the opposite phenotype and enhanced growth factor-mediated signalling in osteoblasts, thereby representing a gain-of-function model for ucOC [6, 7, 36].

Subsequent studies have highlighted that ucOC stimulates insulin gene expression [13] and functions as an insulin secretagogue [36, 37]. In addition to its effect on pancreatic cells, ucOC indirectly promotes insulin secretion by stimulating the secretion of glucagon-like peptide 1 from the small intestine [38]. This sequential hormonal work initiated by ucOC and then mediated by glucagon-like peptide 1 was proposed to be called a bone gut metabolism flow [36, 39].

To close the loop between bone and the pancreas, two independent groups demonstrated that insulin signalling in osteoblasts increases ucOC [36, 38, 40]. Moreover, infusion of ucOC for 2 weeks improved insulin sensitivity, and further experiments in animal models have demonstrated that insulin signalling in osteoblasts increases bone formation and, most importantly, OC production [36, 40]. Moreover, insulin signalling promotes OC decarboxylation, resulting in the release of circulating ucOC [36, 38].

Therefore, it was suggested that there is a regulatory loop between ucOC and insulin: insulin signalling in osteoblasts—which favours ucOC activity by promoting bone remodelling and, in turn, increases ucOC in the circulation. Increased ucOC levels then promote insulin production, secretion, and insulin sensitivity [36, 38, 40].

Afterwards, the next question centred on the applicability of ucOC's beneficial effects. ucOC administration via various routes to obese or even normal rodent models has been experimented with for eventual therapeutic or preventive effects [16, 36, 41]. Long-term oral administration even reduced adipocyte size in mice [36, 42].

As for the endocrine function of ucOC in humans, the role of OC in energy metabolism and insulin resistance has been examined in some cross-sectional and observational studies [2, 20, 36, 43–47], indicating that serum OC and/or ucOC negatively correlate with blood glucose level, insulin level, insulin resistance, and obesity [2, 20, 36, 43–46] and are positively associated with serum adiponectin and insulin production [21, 36, 43, 45, 47]. The active form of OC has been considered a potentially promising biomarker to classify cardiovascular risk and predict T2D prevalence in the MetSy population, especially for those without prevalent T2D [48].

Results from recent studies have indicated sex differences in the metabolic effect of ucOC, and Yasutake et al. showed a possible sex difference in rodent models in the effect of ucOC on glucose homeostasis [36, 42]. ucOC administered orally improved glucose homeostasis in female mice but did not have the same effect in males by causing glucose and insulin intolerance [36, 42]. In humans, decreased ucOC levels were found to be associated with hyperglycaemia and hyperinsulinemia much more in females than in males during an oral glucose tolerance test [36, 45]. In females with MetSy, increased circulating ucOC was detected with decreased TOC levels, but the same detection was not noted in their male counterparts [36, 49]. The responsibility for this gender difference has been attributed to testosterone. Studies have reported that increased ucOC levels promote testosterone production and secretion in male rodent models [36, 42, 50, 51]. Moreover, in clinical studies involving men with central obesity, TOC levels had a positive correlation with testosterone [36, 52]. The same applies to men with or without T2D [21, 36, 43]. In this study of individuals with obesity or overweight, women had higher levels of ucOC compared to men.

This study confirmed, as in other previous studies, the correlation of ucOC, which is supposed to be the active form of OC, with glucose metabolism, obesity markers, and insulin resistance and highlights that waist/hip ratio can be a predictor of ucOC.

5. Conclusion

In the last few years, a growing number of studies have elucidated the function of the bone as an active endocrine organ and, overall, the existing crosstalk between bone and insulin resistance. In addition to its effect as a possible insulin secretagogue, ucOC regulates overall metabolism and targets various organs and tissues, such as adipocytes, skeletal muscle, and the small intestine. Overall, these effects suggest that OC may play a role in protecting against insulin resistance and T2D.

Research into this area is ongoing, but it suggests that OC might be a target for developing new treatments for insulin resistance and T2D. However, more studies are needed to fully understand the mechanisms and potential therapeutic applications of OC in the treatment of insulin resistance.

This study confirmed that there is a correlation between the suggested active form of OC, ucOC, and insulin resistance as a companion occurrence of overweight and obesity in persons without any medical treatment affecting their OC levels and demonstrated that waist/hip ratio is a reliable measure to predict ucOC level in this population. However, the potential benefits of ucOC as a therapeutic agent for treating insulin resistance and MetSy in humans remain to be elucidated.

Acknowledgements

I acknowledge Bernard Tahirbegolli for their help in the statistical analysis of data for the work.

Conflict of interest

The author declares no conflict of interest.

Note

The study has not been published anywhere, but the data was presented as an abstract at the 30th European Congress of Obesity (2023), in Dublin, Ireland [32].

Author details

Venera Berisha-Muharremi
Faculty of Medicine, University of Prishtina, Prishtina, Kosovo

*Address all correspondence to: venera.berisha@uni-pr.edu

References

[1] O'Neill S, O'Driscoll L. Metabolic syndrome: A closer look at the growing epidemic and its associated pathologies. Obesity Reviews. 2015;**16**:1-12

[2] Ferron M, Lacombe J. Regulation of energy metabolism by the skeleton: Osteocalcin and beyond. Archives of Biochemistry and Biophysics. 2014;**561**:137-146

[3] Zoch ML, Clemens TL, Riddle RC. New insights into the biology of osteocalcin. Bone. 2016;**82**:42-49

[4] Ducy P, Amling M, Takeda S, Priemel M, Schilling AF, Beil FT, et al. Leptin inhibits bone formation through a hypothalamic relay: A central control of bone mass. Cell. 2000;**100**:197-207

[5] Karsenty G. Convergence between bone and energy homeostases: Leptin regulation of bone mass. Cell Metabolism. 2006;**4**:341-348

[6] Berisha-Muharremi V. Osteocalcin and Type 2 Diabetes Mellitus: The Hormonal Role of Osteocalcin in Human Glucose Metabolism. Saarbrücken: Lambert Academic Publishing; 2016

[7] Berisha-Muharremi V. Osteocalcin and type 2 diabetes mellitus [thesis]. University of Zagreb, School of Medicine; 2014. Available from: https://www.repozitorij.mef.unizg.hr/islandora/object/mef:5883/datastream/PDF [Accessed: 5 May 2024]

[8] Lee NK, Sowa H, Hinoi E, Ferron M, Ahn JD, Confavreux C, et al. Endocrine regulation of energy metabolism by the skeleton. Cell. 2007;**130**:456-469

[9] Lee NK, Karsenty G. Reciprocal regulation of bone and energy metabolism. Trends in Endocrinology and Metabolism. 2008;**19**:161-166

[10] Fukumoto S, Martin TJ. Bone as an endocrine organ. Trends in Endocrinology and Metabolism. 2009;**20**:230-236

[11] Motyl KJ, McCabe LR, Schwartz AV. Bone and glucose metabolism: A two-way street. Archives of Biochemistry and Biophysics. 2010;**503**:2-10

[12] Lee AJ, Stephen H, Richard E. Measurement of osteocalcin. Annals of Clinical Biochemistry. 2000;**37**:4332-4446

[13] Hauschka PV, Lian JB, Cole DE, Gundberg CM. Osteocalcin and matrix Gla protein: Vitamin K-dependent proteins in bone. Physiological Reviews. 1989;**69**:990-1047

[14] Ducy P, Desbois C, Boyce B, Pinero G, Story B, Dunstan C, et al. Increased bone formation in osteocalcin-deficient mice. Nature. 1996;**382**:448-452

[15] Otabe S, Yuan X, Fukutani T, Wada N, Hashinaga T, Nakayama H, et al. Overexpression of human adiponectin in transgenic mice results in suppression of fat accumulation and prevention of premature death by high-calorie diet. American Journal of Physiology. Endocrinology and Metabolism. 2007;**293**:E210-E218

[16] Ferron M, Hinoi E, Karsenty G, Ducy P. Osteocalcin differentially regulates beta cell and adipocyte gene expression and affects the development of metabolic diseases in wild-type mice. Proceedings of the National Academy of Sciences of the United States of America. 2008;**105**:5266-5270

[17] Kindblom JM, Ohlsson C, Ljunggren O, Karlsson MK, Tivesten A, Smith U, et al. Plasma osteocalcin is inversely related to fat mass and plasma glucose in elderly Swedish men. Journal of Bone and Mineral Research. 2009;**24**:785-791

[18] Pittas AG, Harris SS, Eliades M, Stark P, Dawson-Hughes B. Association between serum osteocalcin and markers of metabolic phenotype. The Journal of Clinical Endocrinology and Metabolism. 2009;**94**:827-832

[19] Im JA, Yu BP, Jeon JY, Kim SH. Relationship between osteocalcin and glucose metabolism in postmenopausal women. Clinica Chimica Acta. 2008;**396**:66-69

[20] Fernández-Real JM, Izquierdo M, Ortega F, Gorostiaga E, Gómez-Ambrosi J, Moreno-Navarrete JM, et al. The relationship of serum osteocalcin concentration to insulin secretion, sensitivity, and disposal with hypocaloric diet and resistance training. The Journal of Clinical Endocrinology and Metabolism. 2009;**94**:237-245

[21] Kanazawa I, Yamaguchi T, Yamamoto M, Yamauchi M, Kurioka S, Yano S, et al. Serum osteocalcin level is associated with glucose metabolism and atherosclerosis parameters in type 2 diabetes mellitus. The Journal of Clinical Endocrinology and Metabolism. 2009;**94**:45-49

[22] Zhou M, Ma X, Li H, Pan X, Tang J, Gao Y, et al. Serum osteocalcin concentrations in relation to glucose and lipid metabolism in Chinese individuals. European Journal of Endocrinology. 2009;**161**:723-729

[23] Winhofer Y, Handisurya A, Tura A, Bittighofer C, Klein K, Schneider B, et al. Osteocalcin is related to enhanced insulin secretion in gestational diabetes. Diabetes Care. 2010;**33**:139-143

[24] Kanazawa I, Yamaguchi T, Yamauchi M, Yamamoto M, Kurioka S, Yano S, et al. Adiponectin is associated with changes in bone markers during glycemic control in type 2 diabetes mellitus. The Journal of Clinical Endocrinology and Metabolism. 2009;**94**:3031-3037

[25] Okazaki R, Totsuka Y, Hamano K, Ajima M, Miura M, Hirota Y, et al. Metabolic improvement of poorly controlled noninsulin-dependent diabetes mellitus decreases bone turnover. The Journal of Clinical Endocrinology and Metabolism. 1997;**82**:2915-2920

[26] Berisha-Muharremi V, Kusec V, Kolaric B, Pavlic-Renar I. Undercarboxylated osteocalcin in patients with newly diagnosed type 2 diabetes after blood glucose regulation. Polish Archives of Internal Medicine. 2018;**128**(3):192-194

[27] Rosato MT, Schneider SH, Shapses SA. Bone turnover and insulin-like growth factor I levels increase after improved glycemic control in noninsulin-dependent diabetes mellitus. Calcified Tissue International. 1998;**63**:107-111

[28] Prats-Puig A, Mas-Parareda M, Riera-Pérez E, González-Forcadell D, Mier C, Mallol-Guisset M, et al. Carboxylation of osteocalcin affects its association with metabolic parameters in healthy children. Diabetes Care. 2010;**33**:661-663

[29] Viswanath A, Vidyasagar S, Sukumar CA. Osteocalcin and metabolic syndrome. Clinical Medicine Insights: Endocrinology and Diabetes. 2023;**16**:1-7

[30] Zimmermann S, Costa MBW, Mathew A, Krishnan S, Schneider JG, Roomp K, et al. Osteocalcin is independently associated with C-reactive protein during lifestyle-induced weight loss in metabolic syndrome. Metabolites. 2021;**11**(8):526

[31] Ugurlu I, Akalin A, Yorulmaz G. The association of serum osteocalcin levels with metabolic parameters and inflammation in postmenopausal women with metabolic syndrome. Metabolic Syndrome and Related Disorders. 2022;**20**(4):219-223

[32] Berisha-Muharremi V, Tahirbegolli B, Sopa D, Rexhepi A, Luzha A. Communication between adipose tissue and bone: Waist/hip ratio is a significant predictor of undercarboxylated osteocalcin in obesity. [Congress Abstract]. Obesity Facts. 2023;**16**(S1):109. DOI: 10.1159/000530456

[33] World Health Organisation. Obesity and overweight. [Internet]. Available from: https://www.who.int/news-room/fact-sheets/detail/obesity-and-overweight#:~:text=children%20and%20adolescents.Adult,than%20or%20equal%20to%2030 [Accessed: 20 March 2024]

[34] Matthews DR, Hosker JP, Rudenski AS, Naylor BA, Treacher DF, Turner RC. Homeostasis model assessment: Insulin resistance and beta-cell function from fasting plasma glucose and insulin concentrations in man. Diabetologia. 1985 Jul;**28**:412-419

[35] Radcliffe Department of Medicine. HOMA calculator. [Internet]. Available from: https://www.dtu.ox.ac.uk/homacalculator/ [Accessed: 20 March 2024]

[36] Mizokami A, Kawakubo-Yasukoch T, Hirata M. Osteocalcin and its endocrine functions. Biochemical Pharmacology. 2017;**132**:1-8. DOI: 10.1016/j.bcp.2017.02.001

[37] Hinoi E, Gao N, Jung DY, Yadav V, Yoshizawa T, Myers MG, et al. The sympathetic tone mediates leptin's inhibition of insulin secretion by modulating osteocalcin bioactivity. The Journal of Cell Biology. 2008;**183**:1235-1242

[38] Ferron M, Wei J, Yoshizawa T, Del Fattore A, DePinho RA, Teti A, et al. Insulin signaling in osteoblasts integrates bone remodeling and energy metabolism. Cell. 2010;**142**:296-308

[39] Mizokami A, Yasutake Y, Gao J, Matsuda M, Takahashi I, Takeuchi H, et al. Osteocalcin induces release of glucagon-like peptide-1 and thereby stimulates insulin secretion in mice. PLoS One. 2013;**8**:e57375

[40] Fulzele K, Riddle RC, DiGirolamo DJ, Cao X, Wan C, Chen D, et al. Insulin receptor signaling in osteoblasts regulates postnatal bone acquisition and body composition. Cell. 2010;**142**:309-319

[41] Ferron M, McKee MD, Levine RL, Ducy P, Karsenty G. Intermittent injections of osteocalcin improve glucose metabolism and prevent type 2 diabetes in mice. Bone. 2012;**50**:568-575

[42] Yasutake Y, Mizokami A, Kawakubo-Yasukochi T, Chishaki S, Takahashi I, Takeuchi H, et al. Long-term oral administration of osteocalcin induces insulin resistance in male mice fed a high-fat, high-sucrose diet. American Journal of Physiology. Endocrinology and Metabolism. 2016;**310**(8):E662-E675. DOI: 10.1152/ajpendo.00334.2015

[43] Buday B, Pach FP, Literati-Nagy B, Vitai M, Vecsei Z, Koranyi L. Serum

osteocalcin is associated with improved metabolic state via adiponectin in females versus testosterone in males. Gender specific nature of the bone-energy homeostasis axis. Bone. 2013;**57**:98-104

[44] Chen X, Wu Y, Liu L, Tian H, Yu X. Osteocalcin is inversely associated with glucose levels in middle-aged Tibetan men with different degrees of glucose tolerance. Diabetes/Metabolism Research and Reviews. 2014;**30**:476-482

[45] Kanazawa I, Yamaguchi T, Tada Y, Yamauchi M, Yano S, Sugimoto T. Serum osteocalcin level is positively associated with insulin sensitivity and secretion in patients with type 2 diabetes. Bone. 2011;**48**:720-725

[46] Chen L, Li Q, Yang Z, Ye Z, Huang Y, He M, et al. Osteocalcin, glucose metabolism, lipid profile and chronic low-grade inflammation in middle-aged and elderly Chinese. Diabetic Medicine. 2013;**30**:309-317

[47] Lacombe J, Karsenty G, Ferron M. *In vivo* analysis of the contribution of bone resorption to the control of glucose metabolism in mice. Molecular Metabolism. 2013;**2**:498-504

[48] Riquelme-Gallego B, García-Molina L, Cano-Ibáñez N, Sánchez-Delgado G, Andújar-Vera F, García-Fontana C, et al. Undercarboxylated osteocalcin: A promising target for early diagnosis of cardiovascular and glycemic disorders in patients with metabolic syndrome: A pilot study. Nutrients. 2022;**14**:2991

[49] Liu JJ, Toy WC, Wong MDS, Tan CSH, Tavintharan S, Wong MS, et al. Elevated undercarboxylated and reduced carboxylated osteocalcin are associated with metabolic syndrome in middle age Asian females. Experimental and Clinical Endocrinology & Diabetes. 2013;**121**:329-333. DOI: 10.1055/s-0033-1334883

[50] Oury F, Sumara G, Sumara O, Ferron M, Chang H, Smith CEE, et al. Endocrine regulation of male fertility by the skeleton. Cell. 2011;**144**:796-809. DOI: 10.1016/j.cell.2011.02.004

[51] Oury F, Ferron M, Huizhen W, Confavreux C, Xu L, Lacombe J, et al. Osteocalcin regulates murine and human fertility through a pancreas-bone-testis axis. The Journal of Clinical Investigation. 2013;**123**:2421-2433. DOI: 10.1172/JCI65952

[52] Liao M, Guo X, Yu X, Pang G, Zhang S, Li J, et al. Role of metabolic factors in the association between osteocalcin and testosterone in Chinese men. The Journal of Clinical Endocrinology and Metabolism. 2013;**98**:3463-3469. DOI: 10.1210/jc.2013-1805

Chapter 7

Stress-Induced Insulin Resistance: Role of Von Willebrand Factor

Gausal A. Khan, Anish Murtaja Alam Khan, Bandana Singh and Mohammed Eid Alqahtani

Abstract

Sterile inflammation (SI) is a non-pathogen-induced inflammation where damage-associated molecular patterns (DAMPs) molecules are released from dying cells, which activate Toll-like receptors (TLRs), leading to insulin resistance (IR) and CVDs. The relationship between inflammation and IR is known. However, the role of SI molecules, that is, HMGB1 and circulating nucleic acids (CNAs), [i.e., eRNA and eDNA], in the development of IR is not known. Glucose intolerance is a fundamental clinical characteristic of metabolic syndrome, which is increasingly prevalent and causing illness globally. Hypoxia resulting from various respiratory disorders often coincides with heightened sympathetic activity, poor nitric oxide (NO) production, and insulin resistance (IR). However, the molecular mechanism remains obscure. Therefore, we hypothesized that SI molecules released during stress might impair NO production and IR. We have shown that stress induces the SI molecule (HMGB1), inhibits insulin-induced NO production, and exerts IR through von Willebrand factor (vWF). The putative vWF sequence could be used as a therapeutic drug for the treatment of IR in the future. These data may have important implications for glucose metabolism in patients with disorders characterized by stress-induced IR.

Keywords: stress, nitric oxide (NO), hypoxia, von Willebrand factor (vWF), high-mobility group box protein 1 (HMGB1), sterile inflammation (SI), circulating nucleic acids (CNAs), insulin resistance (IR), damage-associated molecular patterns (DAMPs), extracellular RNA (eRNA), extracellular DNA (eDNA)

1. Introduction

Inflammation, a natural reaction to adverse stimuli, is essential for health but can lead to diseases if not well controlled. It appears in two primary forms: acute, which is short term, and chronic, which is long lasting and may be associated with disorders. Hypoxia, which is oxygen deprivation, is a non-microbial stimulus that can cause inflammation and stimulate the immune system. Damage-associated molecular patterns (DAMPs) are released as part of this response. These DAMPs interact with certain receptors and start pro-inflammatory pathways. Hypoxia is linked to insulin resistance, a state in which cells become less sensitive to insulin, resulting in disrupted glucose metabolism. It is essential to comprehend the mechanisms that cause inflammation and insulin resistance due to low oxygen levels in order to create successful treatments. Hypoxia is a distinct form of stress that triggers the release of DAMPs and stimulates the innate immune system, resulting in various disease pathways. The production of damage-associated molecular patterns (DAMPs) due to stress triggers Toll-like receptors (TLRs) or RAGE, resulting in inflammatory reactions, leukocyte adhesion, thrombosis, and insulin resistance (IR). Endothelial dysfunction (ED) can be caused by hypoxia or hypoxic stress. This can cause the production of more multimeric von Willebrand factor (vWF). This decrease in nitric oxide (NO) production in the body might enhance IR. We have discussed the role of vWF in the development of IR in animal models.

IR plays a crucial role in the onset of many metabolic and cardiovascular diseases, which are collectively referred to as the metabolic syndrome. Recent studies have demonstrated a connection between IR and ED in relation to CVDs, such as hypertension, coronary artery disease, and atherosclerosis. ED is associated with decreased vasodilation and unexpected vasoconstriction when exposed to NO-releasing stimuli. This condition is strongly related to insufficient endothelial-derived NO, which is considered the main factor connecting IR and ED.

This chapter explains how stress led to sterile inflammation, which then resulted in IR in an animal model. We elaborated on the involvement of vWF in the development of IR and discussed prospective strategies for its prevention.

2. Sterile inflammation (SI)

The body's normal response to harmful stimuli, which can include pathogens, irritants, or damaged cells, is inflammation. Redness, pain, heat, swelling, and loss of function are some of the symptoms. It is a protective mechanism that keeps harmful stimuli out of the body and starts the healing process. Inflammation is primarily categorized into two main types: *acute and chronic inflammation*. *Acute inflammation* is a short-term response that typically lasts for a few days, whereas *chronic inflammation* persists for months or even years and may be associated with various diseases [1]. Another classification distinguishes between sterile inflammation (SI) and non-sterile inflammation (non-SI). In SI, the immune response is triggered against non-microbial antigens, such as drugs, burns, cancer, and autoimmune diseases. Conversely, in non-SI, the immune response is directed against microbial antigens [1–3].

In sterile inflammation (SI), the inflammatory response mirrors that of a non-sterile infection when a pathogen is present. It is characterized by the recruitment of macrophages and neutrophils, the production of reactive oxygen species (ROS), and the activation of proteases. Much like inflammation seen in infections, SI also induces the release of pro-inflammatory cytokines and chemokines. The onset of inflammation in SI is triggered by alterations or misplacement of normal cells, causing the immune system's self-molecules to generate a damage signal referred to as damage-associated molecular patterns (DAMPs) [2]. Normally, DAMPs are endogenous factors situated within cells, hidden from the immune system. However, during injury or cellular stress, dying cells release DAMPs into the extracellular environment, initiating inflammation upon interaction with their receptors (**Table 1**) under sterile conditions. Various DAMPs serve as SI signals associated with specific pathological conditions, earning them the designation of SI markers [4]. These are discussed below.

DAMPs	Putative sensor
HMGIVI	TLR2, TLR4, TLR9, RAGE, CD24
HSP	TLR2, TLR-4, CD91, CD24, CD14, CD-40
S100 proteins	TER2, TLR4, RAGE
RNA	TLR3
DNA	TLR9, AIM2
mtDNA	TLR9
Chromogranin A	NLRP3, NLRPI, CD36, CD14, TLR2, RAGK TLR, NLRPS, RAGE

Table 1.
DAMPs and their receptors of the SI markers are elaborated in brief.

2.1 Circulating nucleic acids (CNAs)

When the body experiences tissue damage or vascular injury, certain materials such as nucleic acids and histones leak out. These substances, when they come into contact with cells lining blood vessels and circulating in the bloodstream, can contribute to the body's defense mechanisms, particularly inflammation. This suggests that extracellular nucleic acids play a role in our natural immunity and support the healing of wounds [5]. Different types of extracellular RNA (eRNA) have distinct effects on the structure and protective function of the blood vessel lining. For example, ribosomal RNA (rRNA) appears to stimulate cytokines, causing increased permeability, while microRNA (miRNA) influences stability. Viral RNAs are also detected by Toll-like receptors (TLRs). Moreover, mitochondrial DNA (mtDNA) is identified as a signaling factor that activates Toll-like receptor 9 (TLR9), interferon gene pathways, and Nod-like receptors, contributing to various immune responses [6]. Extracellular RNA (eRNA) is RNA originating from within the body and is released from dying cells, activating Toll-like receptors (TLRs). eRNA is discharged from stressed or injured cells in various pathological situations. TLR3 not only identifies viral double-stranded RNA (dsRNA) but also self-molecules produced during tissue damage and inflammation, such as eRNA [7]. When TLR3 is activated, the adaptor protein TRIF facilitates a response that involves the activation of interferon (IFN) regulatory factor-3 (IRF-3). IRF-3, in turn, triggers the expression of primary genes, including IFN-β. This secreted IFN-β then participates in either autocrine or paracrine signaling, leading to the production of secondary genes involved in antiviral and antimicrobial responses. In this manner, TLR3 can recognize both pathogen-associated molecular patterns (PAMPs) and danger-associated molecular patterns (DAMPs) [8].

2.2 High-mobility group box 1 (HMGB1)

High-mobility group box 1 (HMGB1) is a protein normally found inside cells, where it interacts with DNA and histones, influencing chromatin structure and regulating processes such as transcription. However, when it is exposed outside the cell, it becomes significant in inflammation. HMGB1 plays a crucial role in various diseases, such as rheumatoid arthritis, scleroderma, Behcet's disease, myositis, and more. Numerous pieces of evidence support its importance in immune-mediated diseases, including increased expression in diseased tissue, induction of characteristic tissue pathology, and elevated levels in blood and urine [9]. Outside the cell, extracellular HMGB1 tends to bind with other pro-inflammatory molecules, leading to the activation of pro-inflammatory cytokine production through stimulation of the TLR4 receptor. Although numerous receptors have the ability to bind to the HMGB1 complex, only two receptor systems, namely RAGE and TLR4, have been definitively identified as established HMGB1 receptors [10].

2.3 Von Willebrand factor (VWF)

Von Willebrand factor (vWF) is a large multimeric glycoprotein present in plasma and plays a crucial role in normal hemostasis. In instances of tissue or vascular injury, it acts as a molecular bridge, connecting platelets to subendothelial components [11]. The direct association between vWF and inflammation lies in its ability to recruit leukocytes, either directly or indirectly by first recruiting platelets, which then attract leukocytes. Elevated levels of vWF are observed in inflammatory conditions and diseases such as arthritis, diabetes, and sepsis [12]. Additionally, vWF can oversee the synthesis of Weibel-Palade bodies (WPBs), which contain well-known inflammation contributors such as P-selectin, IL-8, and eotaxin-3 [13]. vWF, a substantial glycoprotein present in plasma, exists in diverse multimeric forms. Its primary function involves facilitating the connection, movement, and eventual attachment of platelets to regions of damaged endothelium, especially under the high shear conditions of arterial blood flow exceeding a critical threshold of 500–1000 s^{-1} [14]. Additionally, vWF plays a role in safeguarding the coagulation factor VIII (FVIII) from swift proteolytic inactivation. This protein is coded distally on chromosome 12's short arm, synthesized by endothelial cells and megakaryocytes. The primary translation product spans 2813 amino acids (AA), encompassing a 22-residue signal peptide, a significant pro-peptide, and the mature subunit consisting of 2050 residues (pre-pro-vWF). The gene, covering 178–180 kb with 52 exons, encodes the vWF monomer with a molecular weight (MW) of 250–270 kDa. This monomer consists of A, B, C, and D-domains, containing binding sites for various proteins.

2.4 Pro-vWF

Molecules form dimers in the endoplasmic reticulum through disulfide bonds near their carboxyl termini ("tail to tail"). Subsequently, vWF dimers are transported to the Golgi apparatus, where they develop into large multimers, reaching sizes up to 20,000 kDa through N-terminal disulfide bridges ("head to head"). Within the Golgi apparatus, the pro-peptide is removed, and glycation processes also occur [15]. Endothelial cells are responsible for producing plasma vWF, with approximately 95% of endothelial vWF molecules being consistently released into the bloodstream, maintaining a plasma concentration of 10 μg/mL (50 nM or roughly 1 IU/mL). The remaining portion is stored either in cytoplasmic granules known as Weible-Palade bodies or in the α-granules of platelets [16]. In response to stimulation, ultra-large vWF stored in granules can be released through a regulated pathway. A systematic diagram of vWF processing is shown in **Figure 1** [17]. After secretion, the sizable vWF multimers undergo a breakdown into smaller variants facilitated by the metalloprotease ADAMTS-13 (a disintegrin and metalloprotease with thrombospondin type 1 motifs). ADAMTS-13 cleaves the peptide bond between Y1,605 and Y1,606 within the A2 domain of vWF. This process generates circulating plasma vWF with varying multimer sizes. The cleavage also results in vWF subunit fragments of 176 and 140 kDa, contributing to the appearance of "satellite bands" flanking the major band on vWF multimer gels [18]. The role of vWF in genesis of different diseases is as below:

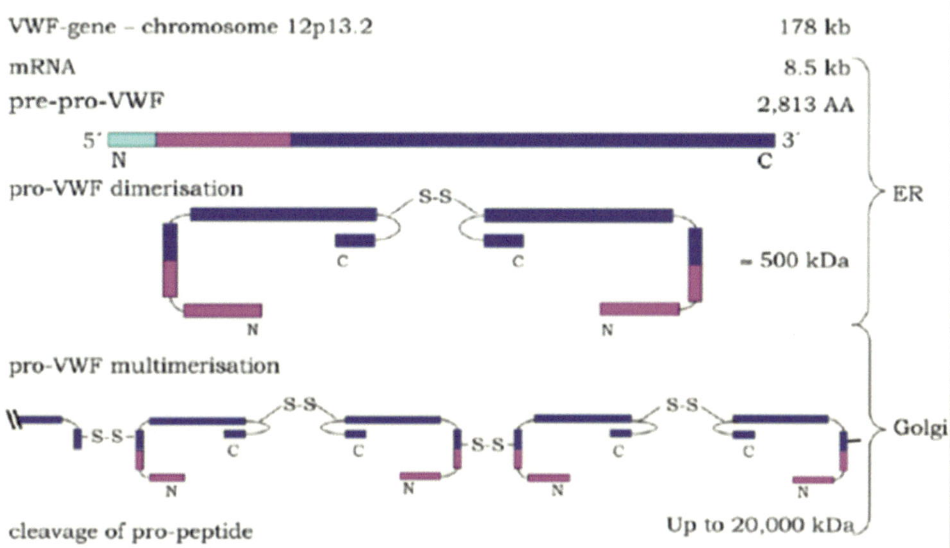

Figure 1.
vWF processing schematic diagram. A signal peptide, a big pro-peptide, and the mature component (pre-pro-vWF) make up the 2813 AA major translation product. In the ER, pro-vWF dimmers' carboxyl termini are where intersubunit disulfide bonds are created. The Golgi apparatus assembles multimers by forming additional intersubunit disulfide bonds close to the mature subunits' amino terminus. After being cleaved off, the pro-peptide remains noncovalently attached to vWF multimers and is concurrently secreted.

2.5 vWF and ischemic heart disease

There is a well-established connection between vWF levels and ischemic heart disease, indicating a potential role for endothelial dysfunction (ED) in the development of coronary artery disease. Individuals who have previously had a heart attack generally have increased levels of von Willebrand factor (vWF) [19]. There is a connection between vWF levels and the intensity of angina symptoms. The fluctuations in vWF levels after acute myocardial infarction have been thoroughly recorded. In a study conducted by Xiang et al. [20] and Geggel et al. [21], it was found that patients who had thrombolytic therapy and were reperfused within 90 minutes experienced a notable 28% rise in vWF levels. These findings indicate that restoring blood flow in cases of acute myocardial infarction may lead to impaired function of the endothelium, causing the release of von Willebrand factor (vWF). Alternatively, reperfusion can remove vWF that was already released from the endothelium or endocardium injured by infarction or ischemia. The release of von Willebrand factor (vWF) in acute myocardial infarction may be associated with the release of free radicals that occur after the infarction and reperfusion process [22]. Higher levels of vWF are associated with a greater likelihood of experiencing another heart attack and a higher chance of death in those with angina and those who have survived a heart attack. A study was conducted to track the progress of 123 individuals who survived a heart attack. The study found that high levels of vWF were identified as separate risk factors for both experiencing another heart attack and death. This is consistent with the results of a previous study, which found that patients who died within a year after experiencing a heart attack had noticeably elevated levels of vWF [23]. The exact mechanism by which elevated vWF increases cardiovascular risk in individuals with angina or post-myocardial-infarction remains unknown. One possibility is that increased endothelial damage in coronary artery disease leads to both heightened thrombin generation and elevated vWF levels. Additionally, it is plausible that vWF may serve as a marker of more severe disease without direct pathophysiological significance (**Figures 2** and **3**).

2.6 vWF and peripheral vascular disease

In patients with peripheral vascular disease, there is a notable elevation in levels of vWF. An illustration of this association comes from the Edinburgh Artery Study, where levels of vWF were significantly higher in 121 study cases compared to matched controls [19]. The heightened levels of vWF in peripheral vascular disease may be attributed to elastase production from activated neutrophils and/or concurrent hypoxia [20].

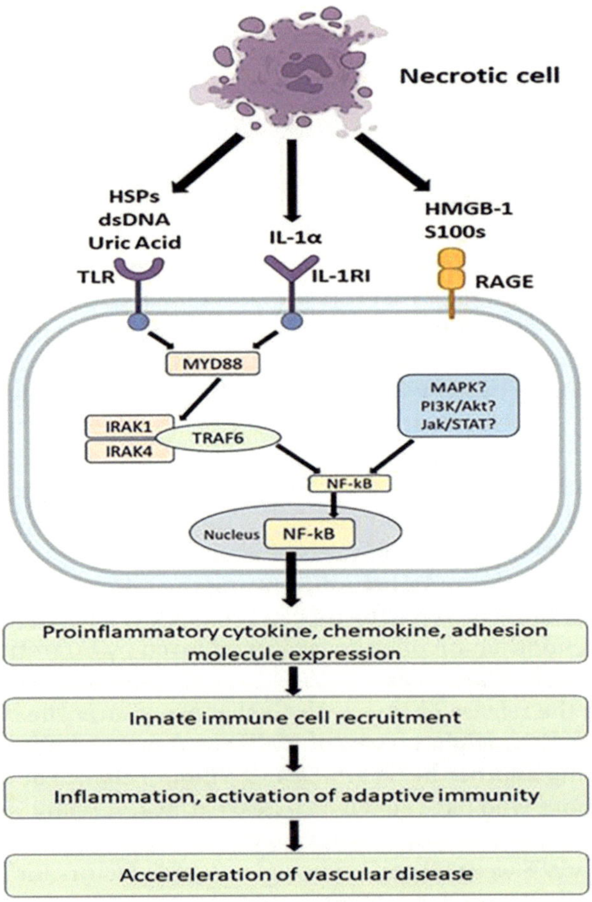

Figure 2.
DAMPs released from necrotic cells ligate cognate or pattern recognition receptors leading to intracellular signaling, gene expression, and inflammation.

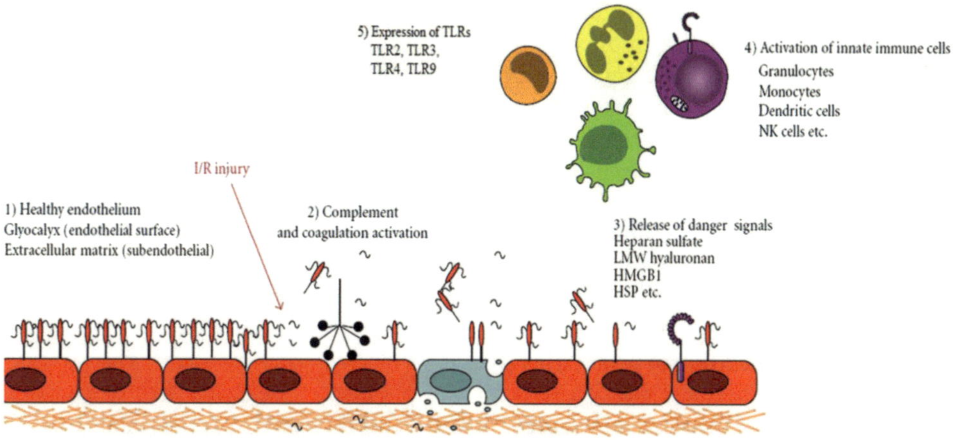

Figure 3.
I-R injury-induced inflammation, coagulation and complement activation, and immune cell recruitment by binding of danger signal via TLR expression.

2.7 vWF and pulmonary vascular disease

The pulmonary vasculature exerts substantial influence on plasma von Willebrand factor (vWF) levels. For example, patients with greater pulmonary vascular resistance and lower cardiac output, regardless of whether they have mitral stenosis or not, have been found to have elevated levels of plasma vWF [24]. Elevated plasma vWF levels are associated with histological evidence of harm to pulmonary endothelial cells in patients with primary pulmonary hypertension. This correlation leads to a higher likelihood of thrombosis, as well as an increase in the release of von Willebrand factor (vWF) from the endothelium due to changes in blood flow dynamics [21].

2.8 vWF in diabetes

Irregularities in von Willebrand factor (vWF) have been detected in diabetes and may contribute to the progression of diabetic vasculopathy [22]. A study conducted by Frankel et al. as part of the Framingham Offspring study demonstrated that elevated levels of vWF were associated with an increased risk of cardiovascular diseases (CVDs) in individuals with type 2 diabetes mellitus or insulin resistance (IR). Moreover, this association was linked to worsened endothelial function and hemostatic imbalance [25]. These findings suggest a potential involvement of vWF in the pathogenesis of cardiovascular complications associated with diabetes.

2.9 vWF and hypertension

As people get older and develop high blood pressure, the natural defenses of the inner lining of blood vessels, called the endothelium, start to weaken. The regulation of blood pressure and cardiovascular hemodynamics is increasingly influenced by changes in vasoactive endothelial factors, including endothelin and prostaglandins [26]. Plasma von Willebrand factor (vWF) can be used as an indicator of endothelial dysfunction or disruption in the context of hypertension, given the documented rise in plasma vWF linked to vascular illness. Patients with hypertension exhibit markedly increased levels of vWF, which tend to return to normal in persons whose hypertension is effectively managed with antihypertensive medications [27]. Elevated concentrations of plasma vWF, fibrinogen, and the soluble adhesion molecule P-selectin (a possible indicator of platelet function) have been detected in individuals with hypertension. Importantly, these marker levels are significantly correlated with diastolic blood pressure levels. However, the levels of these markers were found to be unrelated to whether or not antihypertensive treatment was used or whether good blood pressure control was achieved.

2.10 vWF and inflammatory vascular disease

Patients with inflammatory vascular illnesses and related disorders, including vasculitis, Sjögren's syndrome, Felty's syndrome, giant cell arteritis, and polyarteritis nodosa, have been found to have increased levels of von Willebrand factor (vWF) [24]. Studies examining patients with or without atherosclerosis or connective tissue illness found elevated levels of vWF in all individuals with Raynaud's phenomenon [28]. Individuals diagnosed with systemic sclerosis and Raynaud's phenomenon displayed elevated levels of vWF, especially when diffuse illness was present [29]. These findings suggest a potential association between elevated vWF levels and inflammatory vascular conditions.

2.11 S100B

The S100 protein is part of a family of cytosolic calcium-binding proteins [30]. These proteins play various roles both inside and outside cells, including functions related to apoptosis, inflammation, calcium balance, differentiation, proliferation, migration, and energy metabolism [31]. In cases of acute muscle injury, the regeneration of skeletal muscles relies on appropriate levels of S100B proteins. S100B helps expand the myoblast population and attracts macrophages, promoting a pro-regenerative phenotype and increasing collagen deposition through interactions with FGFR1 (fibroblast growth factor receptor 1) or the RAGE receptor [32]. Additionally, S100B expression is induced in specific cell types when they are activated or undergo neoplastic transformation. Elevated levels of S100B have been reported in conditions such as breast cancer, diabetes, brain injuries, and heart issues [33, 34].

2.12 Heat shock proteins (HSPs)

HSPs are essential proteins found in all cells and are highly conserved. They serve as internal chaperones, playing a crucial role in the folding of proteins and various intracellular processes. When tissues undergo stress due to infection, HSPs trigger the immune system response. They become upregulated during inflammation, activating the immune system by binding to specific Toll-like receptors (TLRs) present on dendritic cells and macrophages. HSPs activate regulatory T cells (Treg) through TLR2 and TLR4, leading to the induction of IL-10 production [35]. Research indicates that the levels of soluble HSP in the bloodstream increase in conditions such as rheumatoid arthritis and juvenile idiopathic arthritis. Besides their immune-stimulating properties, there is evidence supporting an inhibitory role for HSPs in allograft rejection, the activation of autoimmunity, and tumor immunosurveillance [36].

3. Stress

3.1 Types of stress

I. *Acute stress:* This short-term stress occurs in response to immediate challenges or demands. It is a normal part of everyday life and usually subsides once the stressor is removed.

II. *Chronic stress:* This form of stress is chronic and endures for a protracted duration. It might arise from persistent challenges such as work-related troubles, financial struggles, or ongoing health problems.

III. *Episodic acute stress:* This occurs when individuals frequently experience acute stress. People with a tendency to worry excessively or those who lead chaotic, disorganized lives may be prone to episodic acute stress.

IV. *Traumatic stress:* This type of stress results from exposure to a traumatic event, such as a natural disaster, accident, or violent incident. Post-traumatic stress disorder (PTSD) can develop in response to severe traumatic stress. Stress can manifest in various forms, and its impact on human health can be categorized into different types based on their origins and nature. Here are some common types of stress and their physiological, environmental, psychological, and job-related aspects:

3.1.1 Physiological stress

Type: Physical stress on the body, often resulting from illness, injury, or other bodily demands.

Effects: This can lead to increased heart rate, elevated blood pressure, muscle tension, and other physical symptoms. Chronic physiological stress may contribute to the development of various health conditions.

3.1.2 Environmental stress

Type: Arises from external factors in the surroundings, such as noise, pollution, extreme weather conditions, or natural disasters.

Effects: Environmental stress can impact overall well-being, sleep quality, and contribute to the development or exacerbation of respiratory and cardiovascular issues.

3.1.3 Psychological stress

Type: Emotional and mental strain, often resulting from life events, relationships, or personal challenges.

Effects: Psychological stress can lead to anxiety, depression, mood swings, and cognitive difficulties. Chronic psychological stress may also increase the risk of developing mental health disorders.

3.1.4 Job-related stress

Type: Arises from the demands and pressures associated with one's occupation.

Effects: Job-related stress can lead to burnout, fatigue, reduced job satisfaction, and increased risk of physical and mental health issues. Common stressors include tight deadlines, high workload, job insecurity, and conflicts at the workplace.

3.1.5 Social stress

Type: Resulting from interpersonal relationships, social expectations, or societal norms.

Effects: Social stress can impact self-esteem, social interactions, and emotional well-being. Feelings of isolation, loneliness, or societal pressure can contribute to mental health challenges.

3.1.6 Financial stress

Type: Related to economic concerns, such as debt, job insecurity, or financial instability.

Effects: Financial stress can lead to anxiety, sleep disturbances, and impact overall mental health. It may also contribute to physical health issues due to lifestyle changes or inadequate access to healthcare resources.

3.1.7 Coping mechanisms

Type: Adaptive or maladaptive strategies individuals used to deal with stress.

Effects: Healthy coping mechanisms, such as exercise, mindfulness, and social support, can mitigate the impact of stress. Maladaptive coping, such as substance abuse or avoidance, may worsen stress-related health issues.

3.2 Effects of stress on human health

- *Physical health:* Chronic stress is associated with various physical health problems, including cardiovascular issues, high blood pressure, weakened immune system, gastrointestinal problems, and an increased risk of chronic diseases.

- *Mental health:* Prolonged stress can contribute to mental health disorders, such as anxiety and depression. Additionally, it can hinder cognitive abilities, resulting in challenges with focus, relocation, and judgment.

- *Behavioral changes:* People experiencing chronic stress may develop detrimental coping strategies, such as excessive eating, substance misuse, or a sedentary way of life, which can exacerbate health issues.

- *Sleep disturbances:* Stress often disrupts sleep patterns, leading to insomnia or poor-quality sleep. This, in turn, can exacerbate both physical and mental health issues.

- *Emotional impact:* Stress can result in mood swings, irritability, and a reduced ability to manage emotions effectively.

3.3 Here we are discussing about environmental stress such as hypoxic stress

Hypoxia, a condition in which the body lacks oxygen, has a major impact on many cells that are important for vital biological functioning [37]. Oxygen is essential for cellular functions as it acts as the ultimate electron acceptor in the mitochondrial electron transport chain, leading to the production of adenosine triphosphate (ATP) in eukaryotic cells [38].

4. Innate immunity

The innate immune system triggers localized inflammation at the site of initial contact with invading microorganisms or tissue injury. Sterile inflammation is characterized by tissue injury, necrosis, and the release of inflammatory mediators that activate innate immune receptors present in resident macrophages and other immune cells. The concept of pattern recognition receptors (PRRs) was introduced to explain how a limited number of macrophage receptors could bind to a much larger number of bacterial ligands [39]. Damage-associated molecular patterns (DAMPs) provide innocuous signals provided by molecules such as high-mobility group protein B1, uric acid, double-stranded DNA, amyloid-β peptide, heat shock proteins, and IL1α. During necrosis, the loss of plasma membrane integrity allows the release of intracellular materials into the extracellular milieu, stimulating neighboring cells *via* the receptor for advanced glycation end products (RAGE) or Toll-like receptor (TLR). TLRs are recognized as fundamental signaling receptors in the innate immune system, playing a crucial role in activation and initiating inflammatory pathways that lead to the generation of new cytokines and chemokines. Hypoxia-induced cell death and the subsequent release of endogenous ligands from dying cells can activate TLRs [40].

Toll-like receptors (TLRs) play a crucial role in various blood and blood vessel cells, including neutrophils, monocytes/macrophages, and endothelial cells. Human platelets express specific TLRs, such as TLR1, TLR2, TLR4, TLR6, TLR8, and TLR9. TLR2 and TLR4 are associated with inflammatory responses during ischemia-reperfusion injury in the heart [41]. TLR2 has been associated with platelet activation, aggregation, and the formation of platelet-leukocyte aggregates through the PI3K-AKT pathway [42]. TLR4 has been demonstrated to contribute to the early-stage accumulation of foam cells in the intima at sites prone to lesions in the aorta. Systemic administration of the dsRNA analog poly (I:C) (a TLR3 agonist) diminishes neointima formation in a perivascular collar-induced injury model in a TLR3-dependent manner. The expression of TLR9 in platelets induced by oxidative stress has been linked to platelet hyperreactivity, increased aggregation, and thrombosis. TLR signaling proceeds through a sequence of interactions among proteins called adaptor proteins. PAMPs, or pathogen-associated molecular patterns, are specific to groups of microbes and are not found in human cells. DAMPs, or danger-associated molecular patterns, elicit an immune response to trauma, ischemia, cancer, and tissue damage. Inflammatory diseases can lead to increased serum levels of DAMPs [43].

4.1 Endothelial dysfunction in hypoxia

Endothelin-1 acts as a powerful natural constrictor of blood vessels, while nitric oxide (NO) functions as a vasodilator, causing blood vessels to widen [44]. The relationships between different biomarkers have yet to be fully investigated in the challenging conditions of high-altitude environments [45]. In the Mount Everest study, researchers noticed that plasma endothelin-1 (ET-1) levels increased at high altitudes compared to sea level. However, these elevated levels tended to decrease quickly upon descending to lower altitudes [46]. The increased levels of ET-1 in individuals at high altitudes, both patients and healthy individuals, may be due to the hypoxia-induced upregulation of the ET-1 gene expression. Hypoxia also stimulates the activation of genes responsible for producing growth factors for blood vessels and enzymes involved in remodeling. In addition, endothelial dysfunction (ED) involves heightened production of contracting factors from the endothelium, such as angiotensin II and prostanoids. These factors can elevate systemic blood pressure, particularly noticeable at altitudes ranging from 1200 to 3000 meters above sea level [47]. As a result, there is cell growth and inflammation triggered by the activation of nuclear factor-κB (NF-κB), vascular cell adhesion molecule (VCAM), and interleukin-6 (IL-6). VCAM and cytokine activity boost the stickiness of the endothelium, promoting the attachment of inflammatory cells to the endothelial surface. This process leads to vascular inflammation and the formation of blood clots [48]. The study demonstrated a noteworthy increase in serum VCAM-1 levels among both control subjects and patients at high altitudes compared to those at sea level. This elevation was observed in both the high-altitude control group and the patient group, as opposed to the healthy control group at either high altitude or sea level.

5. Hypoxia linked to insulin resistance (IR)

Ascending to high elevations causes a reduction in barometric pressure, which in turn leads to a decrease in the amount of oxygen available. This condition is referred to as "hypobaric hypoxia." Exposure to this stimulus, regardless of its duration, elicits different hormonal reactions, including alterations in insulin signaling, thyroid function, and sympatho-adrenal activity [49]. Hypobaric hypoxia can also impact the gluco-insular axis. Nevertheless, there has been a lack of consistency or agreement in the data. Some research has claimed that hypoxia has favorable effects on peripheral insulin action and body weight regulation [50] while other investigations have reported a degradation of insulin signaling. The Operation Everest II aimed to mitigate the influence of some confounding factors by implementing a consistent ascending profile, food, and exercise regimen throughout a 40-day simulated climb of Mount Everest in a hypobaric chamber. One important discovery was that certain hormonal reactions were more pronounced during the final week of the study when participants were exposed to the lowest level of oxygen concentration [51]. It is worth mentioning that insulin concentrations at the end of the trial were generally twice as high as those at the beginning, while glucose levels remained the same. This indicates the development of insulin resistance. These findings may be significant in understanding how diseases develop at sea level. There is a growing interest in investigating the function of chronic hypoxia as a potential cause of insulin resistance. Chronic intermittent hypoxia (CIH) caused by obstructive sleep apnea (OSA) can potentially contribute to the development and advancement of insulin resistance (IR) and diabetes [52]. Obstructive sleep apnea (OSA) seems to be a factor that can predict impaired glucose metabolism in obese people who are chronically sleep-deprived.

6. Inhibition of nitric oxide production by vWF during hypoxic stress

6.1 Hypoxia-induced vWF inhibits NO synthesis and promotes IR

Chapter 5 as well as earlier studies showed that exposure to hypoxia reduces NO production *in vivo* [53]. However, the mechanism of inhibition of NO synthesis *in vivo* is not clearly understood. Experiments were carried out to investigate the potential involvement of vWF in the suppression of insulin-induced NO generation and the promotion of IR activation. The study revealed that the inclusion of plasma from animals subjected to hypoxia and h-vWF in the reaction mixture hinders the formation of NO caused by insulin (**Figure 4A**). To establish the role of vWF, we used vWF-immunodepleted plasma in the same reaction mixture. The result showed that immunodepletion failed to inhibit insulin-induced NO synthesis (**Figure 4A**).

In order to confirm the inhibitory effect of vWF on insulin-induced NO synthesis, we measured the rate of NO synthesis in the presence of varying concentrations of h-vWF (ranging from 60 to 1000 pM) in the reaction mixture. The findings demonstrated that prior exposure of the reaction mixture to h-vWF effectively suppressed the insulin-induced production of NO in a way that was dependent on the dosage, as depicted in (**Figure 4B**). The most effective suppression was observed at a vWF concentration of 125 pM. Based on this outcome, we utilized a concentration of 125

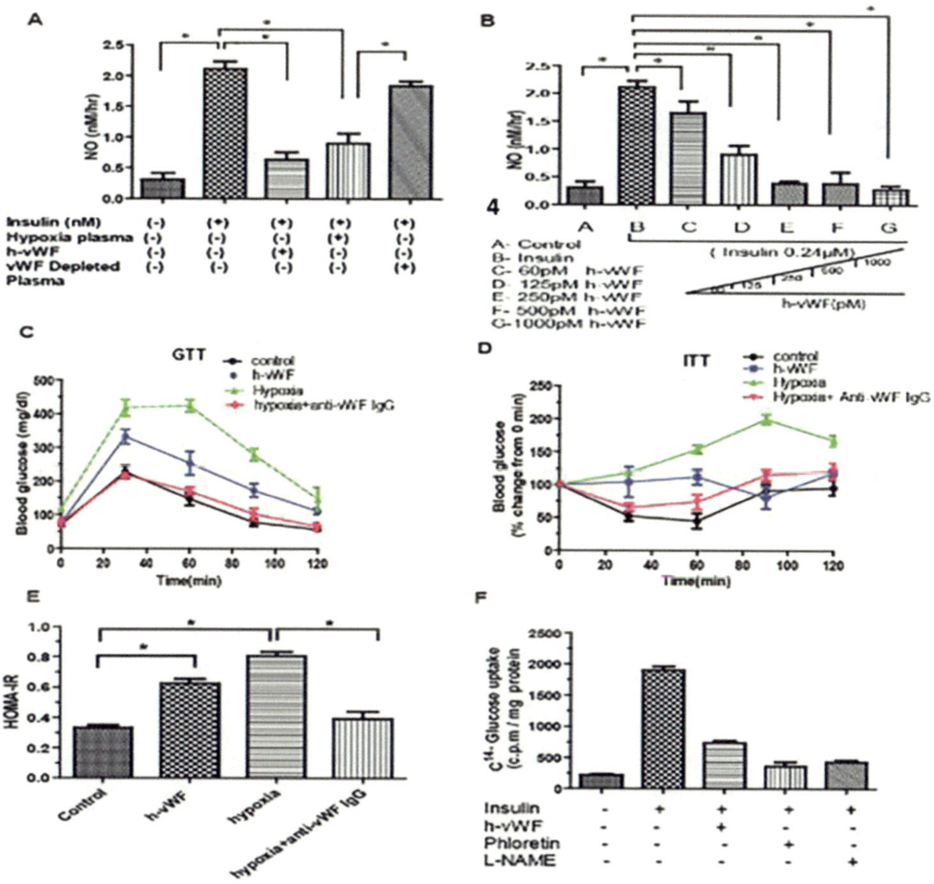

Figure 4.
*A key function of vWF is to limit glucose hemostasis and insulin-induced NO production. (A) The addition of vWF-immunodepleted plasma to the reaction mixture restored the insulin-induced NO generation, while the inclusion of plasma from animals exposed to hypoxia for 24 hours reduced the production of NO. (B) The addition of different doses of h-vWF to the reaction mixture inhibits insulin-induced NO production dose-dependently. (C–E) GTT, ITT, and HOMA-IR in hypoxia/h-vWF as well as anti-neutralizing antibody (2 hours before) infused in mice (n = 4 per group). (F) The uptake of D-[U-14C] glucose by insulin was measured in RBCs pretreated with either h-vWF, phloretin, or L-NAME. Data are means ± SEM of three separate experiments. The results show a significant (*p < 0.05) difference between different time points using one-way ANOVA. Reprinted (adapted) with permission from Ref. [54]. Copyright 2013 American Chemical Society.*

picomolar (pM) von Willebrand factor (vWF) in future experiments. These findings indicate that vWF functions as a suppressor of insulin-induced NO production.

It has been established that insulin-induced glucose uptake is mediated through NO, a second-messenger molecule of insulin [55]. The involvement of vWF in IR has been shown previously [56].

In order to assess the potential impact of von Willebrand factor (vWF) on insulin resistance (IR) caused by the inhibition of nitric oxide synthase (NOS), we conducted several experiments, including glucose tolerance test (GTT), insulin tolerance test (ITT), homeostatic model assessment of insulin resistance (HOMA-IR), and glucose uptake tests on animals, that were either exposed to hypoxia or treated with h-vWF. Animals that were subjected to hypoxia or h-vWF showed a higher susceptibility to insulin resistance (IR), as indicated by the increased glucose tolerance test (GTT) (**Figure 4C**), insulin tolerance test (ITT) (**Figure 4D**), and homeostatic model assessment of insulin resistance (HOMA-IR) scores (**Figure 4E**), as well as a lower level of D-[U-14C] glucose uptake (**Figure 4F**). Conversely, administering a vWF immunoneutralizing antibody 2 hours before hypoxia exposure prevented the inhibitory impact of vWF on glucose metabolism (**Figure 4C–E**). Surprisingly, the neutralization of vWF by antibody did not change the bleeding time (BT) or clotting time (CT). These findings indicate that vWF hinders the generation of NO and the functioning of insulin in inducing insulin resistance.

6.2 NO in hypoxia-induced IR

Subsequent tests were carried out to reaffirm the function of nitric oxide (NO) in ischemia-reperfusion (IR) caused by hypoxia. We performed a series of trials where we administered nitroglycerine (NG) patches transdermally to mice, mimicking the effects of NO. The results of our study show that the use of NG patches applied to the skin effectively prevents hypoxia-induced insulin resistance. This was observed by several tests, including glucose tolerance test (GTT), as shown in **Figure 5A**, insulin tolerance test (ITT) shown in **Figure 5B**, and homeostatic model assessment of insulin resistance (HOMA-IR) shown in **Figure 5C**. Conversely, the administration of the NO inhibitor L-NAME also resulted in insulin resistance, as depicted in **Figure 5A–C**. This observation indicates that the suppression of insulin-induced nitric oxide (NO) generation is responsible for hypoxia-induced insulin resistance (IR).

6.3 Larger doses of insulin prevent vWF-mediated inhibition of insulin-induced NO synthesis

Next, experiments were done to determine if greater doses of insulin can prevent the suppression of insulin-induced NO production by vWF. In our study, we observed that higher concentrations of insulin (ranging from 0 to 1200 nM) in the reaction mixture counteracted the inhibitory impact of vWF in a manner that was dependent on the dosage, as shown in (**Figure 6**). The results indicate that the interaction between insulin and eNOS is hindered by vWF in a competitive manner, leading to the inhibition of NO generation. Put simply, it implies that vWF and insulin vie for the identical binding site of eNOS.

6.4 Binding of vWF to eNOS detected with far-western blotting and CoIP

Based on the aforementioned observations, it may be deduced that vWF indirectly attaches to eNOs and hinders the generation of NO. In order to gain conclusive proof of

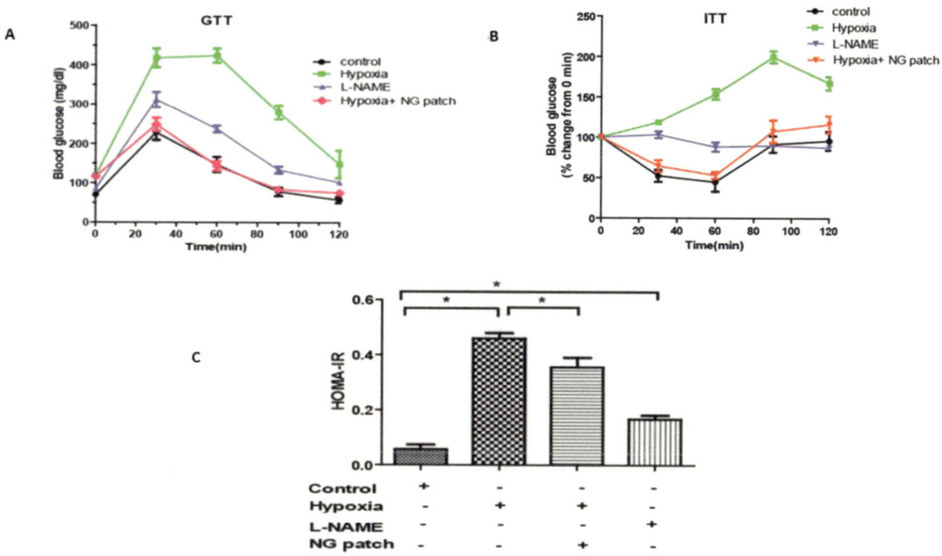

Figure 5.
*In hypoxia, vWF induces IR in a NO-dependent manner. (A) GTT, (B) ITT, and (C) HOMA-IR in control, hypoxia-exposed, L-NAME-treated, and nitroglycerin (NG) patch-treated mice. The application of the NG patch reverses the effects of hypoxia, but the L-NAME (70 mg/kg of body weight) treatment significantly increases GTT, ITT, and HOMA-IR scores. Data are means ± SEM of three separate experiments. The results show a significant (*p < 0.05) difference between different time points using a one-way ANOVA. Reprinted (adapted) with permission from Ref. [54]. Copyright 2013 American Chemical Society.*

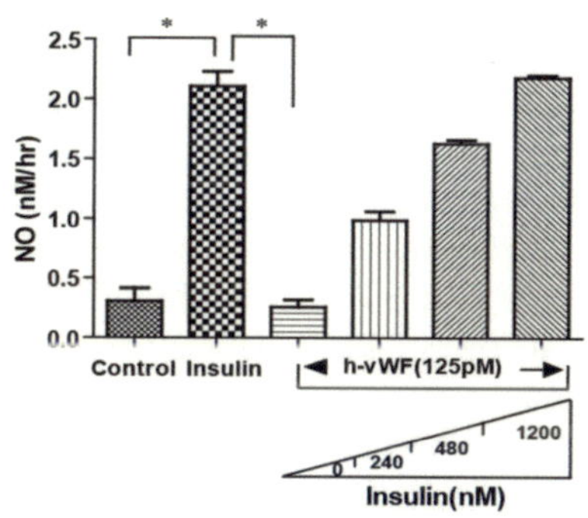

Figure 6.
*vWF-mediated inhibition of NO production reversed by larger doses of insulin. The addition of larger doses of insulin dose-dependently (0–1200 nM) to the reaction mixture eliminates the inhibitory effect of vWF. Data are means ± SEM of triplicate reactions from three separate experiments. The results showed a significant (*p < 0.05) difference in comparison to the control using a one-way ANOVA. Reprinted (adapted) with permission from Ref. [54]. Copyright 2013 American Chemical Society.*

the binding, we initially conducted far-western blotting using RBC membrane lysates that expressed the native eNOS. These lysates acted as the target prey, while the h-vWF protein served as the bait protein. The experimental procedure is described in detail in the materials and methods section. The positive control in this study involved using purified human eNOS protein, while the negative control consisted of ECV-304 cell lysate missing eNOS. The interaction between the prey protein and the bait protein was identified using a particular anti-vWF antibody. Within the lanes containing the RBC membrane lysates and eNOS, h-vWF exhibited binding to a 130 kDa protein, which corresponded to the size of this molecule (**Figure 7A**). The lane containing the ECV-304 cell lysate (negative control) did not show any band detection. Next, the membrane was removed and subsequently probed again using a rabbit monoclonal eNOS antibody. A band with a molecular weight of 130 kDa was observed in both lanes, specifically in the ones containing the red blood cell membrane lysate and endothelial nitric oxide synthase (eNOS) (**Figure 7B**). The lane containing the ECV-304 cell lysate did not exhibit any discernible band. Collectively, our findings demonstrated the precise interaction between vWF and eNOS present in both RBC cells and the cell-free system.

To revalidate the far-western blotting result, we performed CoIP experiments, eNOS was immunoprecipitated by vWF and the subsequent vWF antibody from RBC membrane lysates (experimental), purified eNOS (positive control), and ECV-304 cell lysate (negative control) detailed in materials and methods. The immune complexes were resolved by SDS-PAGE and immunoblotted for eNOS protein. **Figure 7C** again shows clearly identical bands of 130 kDa in the lanes containing RBC membrane lysate and purified eNOS, but no band was seen in ECV-304 cell lysate, proving that eNOS co-immunoprecipitated with vWF.

In another experiment, we immunoprecipitated vWF from hypoxia-exposed animal plasma (experimental) and h-vWF (positive control) by purifying eNOS protein and immunoblotted the samples for vWF. The results showed that vWF immunoprecipitated with eNOS, that is, the 180 kDa band of vWF was detected in hypoxia-exposed plasma(experimental) and h-vWF (positive control) (**Figure 7D**). However, in the case of vWF, the same molecular mass band was noted (**Figure 7D**). These results further confirm the specific binding of vWF to eNOS in RBCs.

6.5 Determination of KD by SPR

Figure 8 shows the sensogram for the binding of the analyte (h-vWF) at varying concentrations to immobilized human eNOs or mouse eNOS protein on the CM5 sensor chip. The change in the response units with varying ligand concentration indicated the change in the bound mass on eNOS immobilized on the chip (sensor surface) over time. The binding of h-vWF to human eNOS was the strongest because of the faster "on" rate (association constant) ($K_A = 5.6 \times 10^7$ M) as well as the slower "off" rate (dissociation constant) [$K_D = 1.79 \times 10^{-8}$ M (**Figure 8A**)]. On the other hand, the binding of h-vWF to mouse eNOS was also the same [K_A of 5.62×10^7 M and K_D of 1.75×10^{-8} M (**Figure 8B**)]. These data suggest that h-vWF binds either human or mouse eNOS with the same affinity.

6.6 Kinetic analysis of NO production

The kinetic mechanisms of eNOS (enzyme), insulin (activator), and vWF (inhibitor) were assessed by varying the concentrations of insulin and h-vWF. The competitive kinetic constant of vWF was calculated using GraphPad Prism version 5.0. A linearized analysis of the data (Michaelis-Menten equation) revealed a competitive mode of inhibition (**Figure 9A**). By using the double-reciprocal plot, the values of $1/K_m$ and $1/V_{max}$ were quantified; the former increased in the presence of vWF, while the latter remained unchanged, proving the competitive mode of inhibition between the two substrates (**Figure 9B**). We also measured the IC_{50} and K_i value. The IC_{50} and K_i values obtained for vWF were 18.31 pM (**Figure 9C**) and

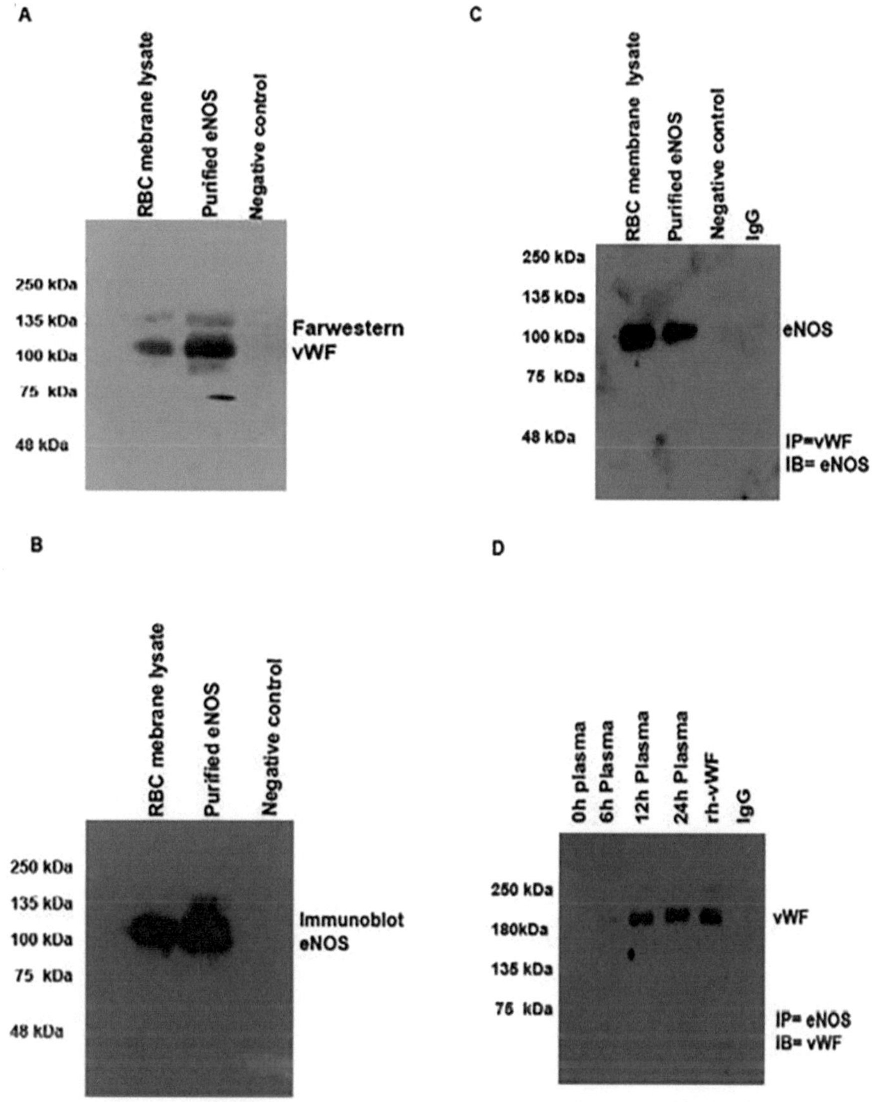

Figure 7.
Far-western blot analysis and CoIP of binding of NOs to vWF. (A) We used purified human eNOS (positive cell-free control), RBC lysate protein (experimental sample), and eNOS-negative ECV-304 cell lysate protein (negative control). The immune-positive bands were detected using the anti-vWF antibody, revealing a 130 kDa band representing the eNOS in both RBC membrane lysate and purified eNOS. (B) the same membrane was striped and reprobed with the anti-eNOS antibody, revealing that of a 130 kDa band. (C) RBC membrane lysate (experimental sample), purified eNOS (positive cell-free control), and ECV-304 cell lysate (negative control) were incubated with h-vWF protein to pull down the eNOS using the anti-vWF antibody. Western blot analysis was performed with the anti-NOS antibody. The detected signals corresponded to the eNOS protein (130 kDa) in both RBC membrane lysate and purified eNOS. No band was observed in ECV-304 cell lysate (negative control). IgG served as the negative control. (D) h-vWF (positive cell-free control) and plasma exposed to hypoxia for different periods of time (experimental samples) were incubated with purified eNOS protein to pull down the vWF using the anti-eNOS antibody. Western blot analysis was performed with the anti-vWF antibody. The detected signals corresponded to the vWF protein (180–150 kDa) in both h-vWF and exposed samples. IgG served as the negative control. These experiments were reproduced thrice. IB, immunoblot; IP, immunoprecipitation. Results are from a representative experiment from three independent experiments. Reprinted (adapted) with permission from Ref. [54]. Copyright 2013 American Chemical Society.

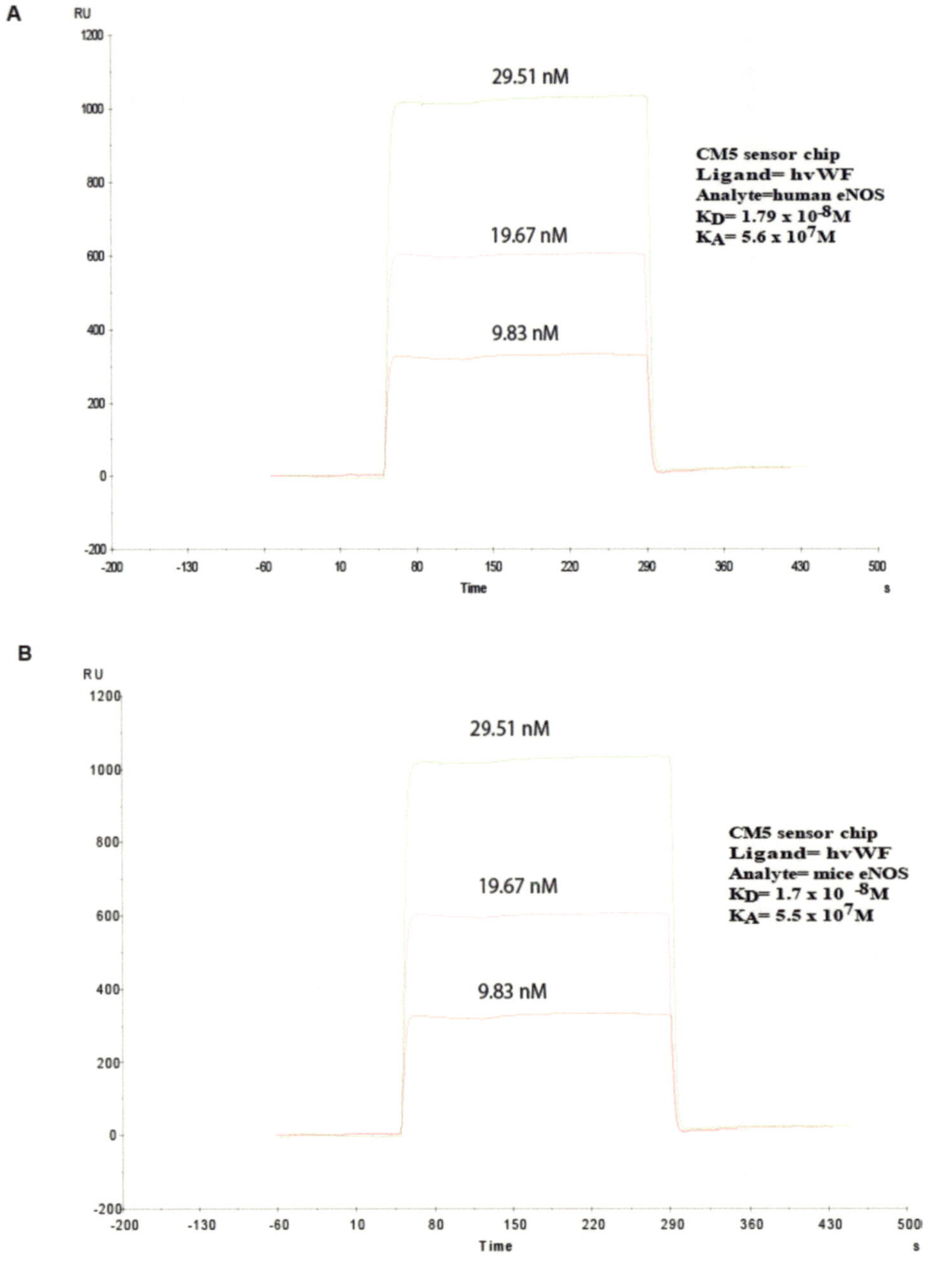

Figure 8.
Surface plasma resonance of binding of vWF to human eNOS or mouse eNOS. Sensorgram showing binding of different concentrations of vWF (9.85, 19.67, and 29.51 nM) immobilized with purified human eNOS or mouse eNOS protein over sensor chip CM5. There is no change in the binding affinity of human vWF with human eNOS or mouse eNOS (RU, response units). Experiments were performed at least three separate times, and typical results are shown. Reprinted (adapted) with permission from Ref. [54]. Copyright 2013 American Chemical Society.

250 pM (**Figure 9D**), respectively. The lower Ki value suggests a higher efficacy of the inhibitor (vWF) for activator (insulin) inhibition. On the other hand, a higher IC_{50} value denotes the higher potency of the inhibitor. The direct plots of reaction velocity

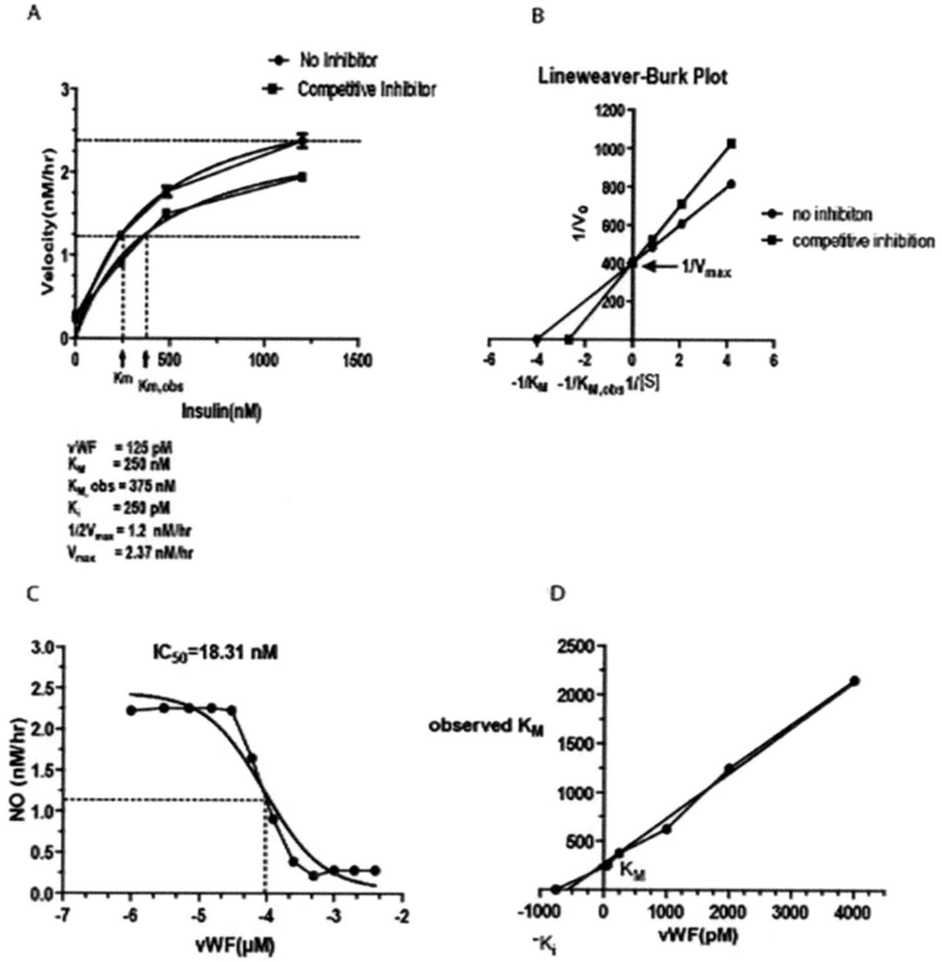

Figure 9.
Enzyme kinetics of eNOS inhibition. (A) Enzyme kinetic analysis of eNOS inhibition by vWF using the Michaelis-Menten equation (B) Lineweaver-Burk plots of reaction velocity vs. substrate concentration for enzyme kinetics of eNOS in the absence and presence of vWF. The values of IC_{50} (C) and Ki (D) for vWF n displacing insulin binding were 18.31 nM and 250 pM, respectively. Results are from a representative experiment from three independent experiments. Experiments were performed at least three separate times, and mean values are shown. All the analysis was done by using the GraphPad Prism version (GraphPad Software, Inc., La Jolla, CA). Reprinted (adapted) with permission from Ref. [54]. Copyright 2013 American Chemical Society.

versus substrate concentration demonstrated classical steady-state kinetic behavior. Best fits for experimental data were assessed by comparison of the standard errors of the mean; nonlinear regression analysis F tests were employed for competitive inhibition fits.

6.7 Determination of vWF-NOS interaction site: *In silico* study vWF (residue 2597 to 2791) a typical member of the cystine-knot family

SWISS molecular modeling of vWF (residue 2597–2791) [57–59] showed high sequence and structural homologs to the "*cystine-knot family*" especially the highly conserved cysteines involved in the formation of the cystine-knot motif

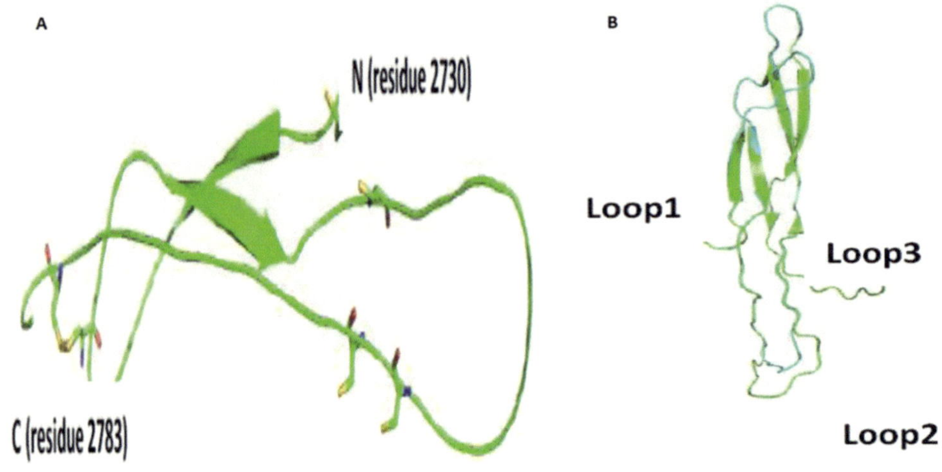

Figure 10.
Insilico modeling of the vWF (residue 2597 to 2791) to determine the vWF-NOS interaction site.

(**Figure 10A**). This region showed high structural homolog to the sclerostin protein known to play a central role in the regulation of bone growth and remodeling [60]. In the entire sequence, only from residue 2730–2783 forming the tertiary structure and the remaining residues were highly unstructured as observed in the sclerostin protein (**Figure 10A–B**).

6.8 The *in silico* molecular simulation

Both vWF (region 2597–2791) (cyan in color) and sclerostin (green in color) superimposed with an RMSD of (0.420 A°) (**Figure 10B**). As per the nomenclature of the cystine-knot family protein, the loop region 2 of vWF differs from sclerostin. In sclerostin, loop 2 is highly perturbed and involved in the interaction with Wnt signaling. The structural as well as sequence similarity of the loop 2 of vWF may also play a crucial functional role in interaction with other proteins.

6.9 Putative interaction of vWF (region 2597–2791) with insulin receptor

A structural modeling study of insulin receptor ecto domains is difficult because of their large size, flexible multi-domain morphology, and extensive glycosylation and disulfide bond poses challenges. The recent crystal structure of insulin receptor ecto domains L1-CR-L-Fn III-1-α CT (04–719) with insulin (the primary binding domain of insulin with a dissociation constant of ~6.4 nm) showed an induced fit. During the fit, α-CT segment displaced on the L1-beta2 structure compared with the apo structure and further confirmed a long-speculated induced fit upon insulin receptor binding [61]. Our experimental study clearly showed that insulin binding was interrupted by the vWF binding. This leads us to develop a valid hypothesis that both (insulin as well vWF) will share common binding sites for their recognition. Assuming this hypothesis, we further propose that the structural region of vWF (region 2730–2783), especially the loop 2 region, may be involved in the binding with the insulin receptor ectodomain region. However, this hypothesis needs to be verified by intensive structural studies.

6.10 Discussion

This study investigated the relationship between increased levels of vWF release and decreased levels of NO production insulin sensitivity during hypoxia.

Here, for the first time, we employ both biochemical and functional methods to demonstrate that vWF serves as a new ligand for eNOS. Von Willebrand factor (vWF) counteracts the effects of insulin, hampers the synthesis of nitric oxide (NO), and induces alterations in glucose regulation. This leads to an increase in the findings of the glucose tolerance test (GTT), insulin tolerance test (ITT), and homeostatic model assessment of insulin resistance (HOMA-IR), as well as a decrease in the rate at which glucose is taken up in an animal model of hypoxia. The binding of vWF to eNOS was demonstrated in RBC membranes and a cell-free system (purified eNOS) by far-western blotting and CoIP. This interaction was also confirmed by SPR in a cell-free system. We further demonstrated that the binding of vWF to eNOs impaired insulin-induced NO production and increased IR; however, larger doses of insulin reversed the inhibitory effect of vWF. Previous studies and also our data suggest that either acute exposure or continuous hypoxia can induce IR. However, the molecular mechanism of IR during hypoxia is still obscure. Previous studies proposed a relationship between CVDs, IR, and ED, where ED has been characterized by an increased rate of vWF release and a decreased level of NO production [62]. Impaired NO production, a phenotype of IR has also been linked to OSA and CVDs [63–65].

Diabetes mellitus and insulin resistance (IR) have also been linked to impaired endothelial function. Treatment with thiazolidinediones, which are insulin sensitizers, has been demonstrated to improve endothelial dysfunction. Our findings also showed that there was an increase in the levels of multimeric forms of vWF in plasma over time, which led to a decrease in NOS activity. We have additionally shown that hypoxic plasma depleted of vWF did not reduce the production of NO generated by insulin. Furthermore, h-vWF also inhibited the production of NO induced by insulin in a manner that depended on the dosage. In contrast, higher dosages of insulin counteracted the effects. On the other hand, the inhibition of vWF by a neutralizing antibody reduced the effects of hypoxia-induced insulin resistance, as shown by the glucose tolerance test (GTT), insulin tolerance test (ITT), and homeostatic model assessment of insulin resistance (HOMA-IR), without affecting the bleeding characteristics. This indicates that vWF may have a significant impact on hypoxia-induced IR by inhibiting NOS and establishing a reverse correlation between vWF and NO production during hypoxia. To reconfirm the role of NO in hypoxia-induced IR, we used NO-mimetic NG patches that were transdermally applied to mice and prevented hypoxia-induced IR. This finding also suggests that hypoxia-induced IR is mediated through inhibition of NO production. To further determine the biological relevance of hypoxia-induced upregulation of vWF and a decreased rate of glucose uptake through NO inhibition, we used h-vWF in our D-[U-^{14}C] glucose uptake assay. Preincubation with either h-vWF or L-NAME completely abrogated insulin-induced glucose uptake in RBCs. In this study, we further demonstrated that the continuous delivery of NO elicited by the application of a transdermal NG patch protected mice from IR. This result suggests that vWF inhibits glucose uptake by inhibiting NO synthesis through inhibition of NOS.

The biological significance of the antagonizing effect of vWF on NO production through direct interaction with NOS is profound. By using far-western blotting, CoIP, and SPR, our study demonstrated for the first time the direct interaction between vWF and NOS. Our data suggest that vWF inhibits insulin-induced NO production by directly binding to eNOS. A previous study had also established that NOS is the receptor, and NO is a second messenger for insulin action [66]. It was also reported that eNOS is a membrane-bound constitutive enzyme whose activation is directly related to the binding of insulin to its specific binding sites on the membrane surface. Here, we performed SPR to determine the affinity of the interaction between vWF and NOS. The resulting sensorgram showed concentration-dependent binding of both molecules, and the affinity of the binding was considerably high, as indicated by a K_D of 1.79×10^{-8}. This finding was further validated by kinetic analyses of both molecules. The results showed a noticeably low inhibitory constant (K_i = 250 pM), as well as IC_{50} (18.31 pM), suggesting a higher affinity of binding to and greater efficacy of inhibition of eNOS by vWF. Under normal conditions, the physiological concentrations of insulin and vWF are 542 and 5.2 nM, respectively [67]. Therefore, vWF never binds to eNOS because the affinity is lower than that of insulin ($K_D = 2.45 \times 10^{-9}$ M). However, under several pathological conditions where the concentration of the ultra large form of vWF is higher than normal [68], insulin-induced NO production is inhibited by the competitive binding of vWF to NOS.

It was also reported that NO has a role in glucose transport and metabolism in rat skeletal muscle through NOS activation [69]. Our results indicate that vWF acts as an inhibitor of NOS and impaired insulin action and NO production. Upon binding to its receptor (NOS), insulin stimulates NO production, which in turn activates the Glut-4 receptor, consequently leading to an increased rate of glucose uptake but a decreased level of platelet aggregation [70]. However, a putative predictive functional region of vWF is shown in (**Figure 10A–B**). However, details of the interaction between the two molecules remain to be explored and the importance of a specific domain and/or sequence of the respective protein still needs to be studied.

This study delineates the mechanism of inhibition of NO production by vWF during hypoxia, where ED is the predominant feature. It might also explain the mechanism of increased IR in patients with CVDs and diabetes mellitus. The data of this study may have important implications for glucose homeostasis at high altitudes and the risk of metabolic diseases for patients with disorders characterized by hypoxia, sleep apnea, and chronic obstructive pulmonary disease.

7. Hypoxia-induced endothelial activation and IR

7.1 Hypobaric hypoxia-induced insulin resistance

Insulin resistance (IR) or glucose intolerance is a fundamental clinical characteristic of metabolic syndrome, a condition whose rising incidence has contributed to heightened cardiovascular morbidity and mortality rates in industrialized nations. The link between IR, cardiovascular diseases, and hypoxia has been noted in various settings, including exposure to high altitudes, hypoxic gas inhalation, or hypobaric conditions, as previously reported in studies involving both human and animal models [71].

We intended to find out whether hypobaric hypoxia has any effect on glucose hemostasis. Animals were exposed to hypoxia and then GTT, ITT, and HOMA-IR values were analyzed. It was found that animals exposed to hypoxia showed time-dependent increases in GTT, ITT, and HOMA-IR values in comparison to those of control animals (**Figure 11A–C**).

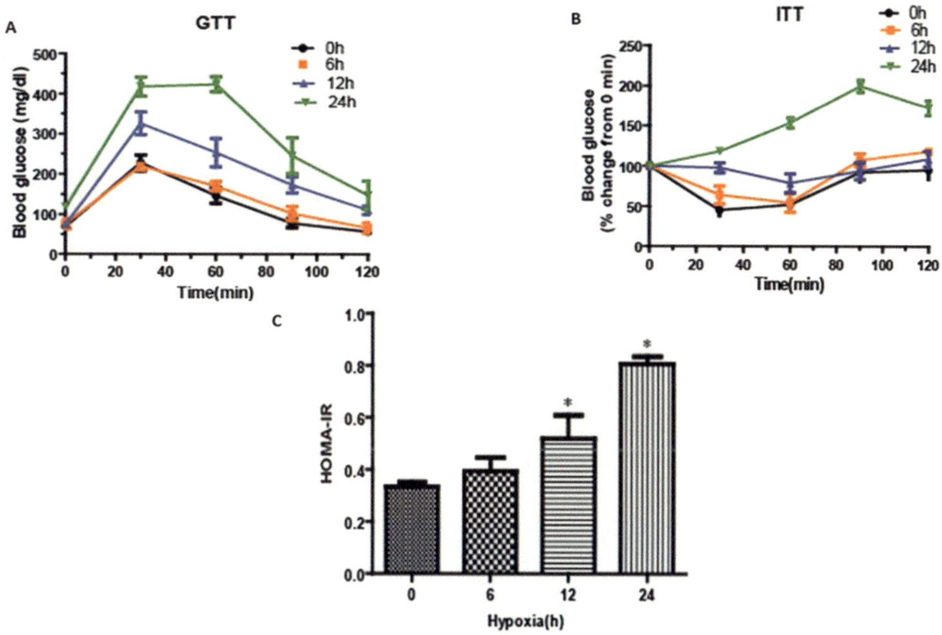

Figure 11.
*Time course study of the effect of hypoxia on glucose metabolism. Animals were exposed to hypoxia as described in materials and methods for 0 (unexposed) 6, 12, and 24 hours. The GTT, ITT, and HOMA-IR were conducted for the IR study. (A) Following a 16-hour fast (n = 4 per group), a glucose tolerance test was conducted. (B) Four mice per group, fed at random and subjected to varying amounts of hypoxia, underwent an insulin tolerance test (0.75 units/kg of insulin). (C) In hypoxia-exposed mice (n = 4 per group), the insulin resistance test was carried out using HOMA-IR scoring. Data are means ± SEM of three separate experiments. The results show a significant (*p < 0.05) difference between different time points using a one-way ANOVA. Reprinted (adapted) with permission from Ref. [54]. Copyright 2013 American Chemical Society.*

7.2 Hypobaric hypoxia-induced endothelial dysfunction

As IR is related to ED. The vascular endothelium produces many substances that contribute importantly to hemostasis and regulation of vessel tone and permeability. Being the largest organ of the body, the endothelium senses any kind of stress and in response, it releases different vasoactive, vasodilator, and inflammatory modulators. Among the two most important molecules, NO and vWF are prominent markers for ED in different pathological conditions, such as chronic pulmonary disease, hypertension, and diabetes mellitus.

To find out the effect of hypobaric hypoxia on NO production, plasma from hypoxia-exposed animals was used in the reaction mixture for identical conditions (**Figure 12A**). Results showed that the addition of insulin to the reaction mixture increases NO production by almost 2.5 nmol/h. On the other hand, the addition of hypoxic plasma to the reaction mixture showed a time-dependent decline in NO production.

Next, we sought to determine whether hypoxia had any role on ED. Decreased NO and increased vWF both are established markers for ED. Mice were exposed to hypoxia for different time intervals (0, 6, 12, 24) hours, with equal numbers of age-matched littermates for each line maintained as control. Plasma was collected for quantifying vWF antigen and NO production. Total vWF:Ag was quantitated by ELISA (**Figure 12B**) and immunoblotting was done from the plasma by using a vWF

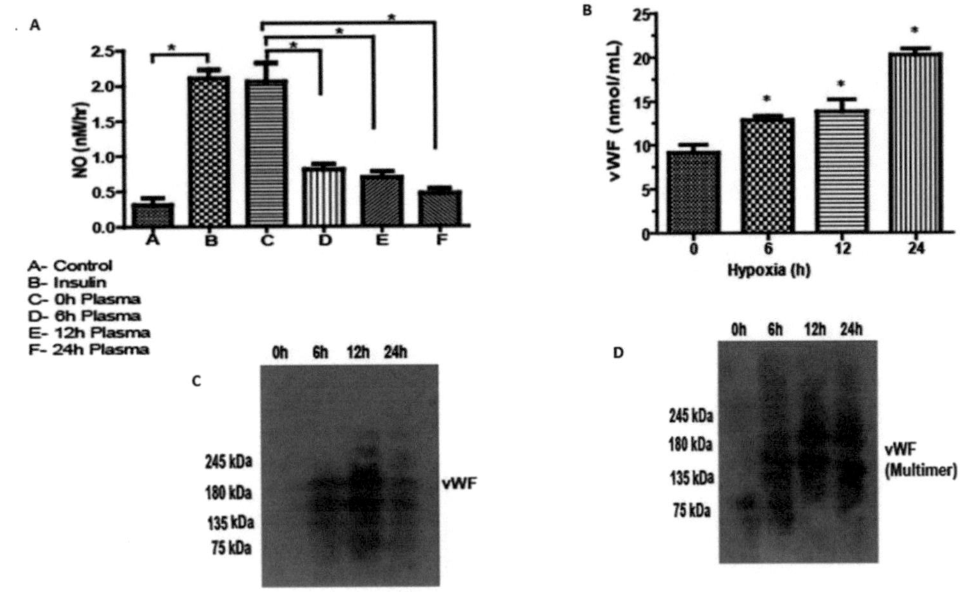

Figure 12.
*Study of the impact of hypoxia on ED over a period of time. According to the instructions in materials and methods, animals were subjected to hypoxia for 0, 6, 12, and 24 hours. For ED, the NO assay, an ELISA of vWF, and SDS immunoblotting were used. (A) Adding plasma from several AH-exposed animals reduced the amount of NO produced by insulin. (B) vWF total antigen quantification in plasma using an ELISA (n = 4 per group). (C) Immunoblotting versus WF at various intervals. (D) Multimer analysis of vWF using immunoblotting at the designated time intervals after SDS-agarose gel electrophoresis. The findings are based on a representative experiment that was conducted three separate times. The three independent experiments' means ± standard error are represented in the data. One-way ANOVA findings indicate a significant (*p < 0.05) difference across time points. Reprinted (adapted) with permission from Ref. [54]. Copyright 2013 American Chemical Society.*

primary antibody. The vWF multimer was analyzed by SDS-agarose PAGE. Gel was transferred to the PVDF membrane and blot with vWF primary antibody. It was seen that hypobaric hypoxia-induced vWF expression increased time-dependently and most of the vWF expressions are multimeric form (**Figure 12C–D**). These results suggest that hypoxia induces ED as well as glucose.

7.3 Discussion

IR is defined as reduced sensitivity and/or responsiveness to the metabolic action of insulin that promotes glucose disposal. It is the fundamental pathophysiologic disturbance responsible for the cluster of metabolic and cardiovascular disorders, collectively known as the metabolic syndrome. In recent years, it has become clear that IR and ED play a central role in the pathogenesis of different disease conditions such as cardiovascular disorders, including hypertension, coronary artery disease, and atherosclerosis. ED is an important component of the metabolic or IR syndrome and this is demonstrated by reduced vasodilation and/or paradoxical vasoconstriction in coronary and peripheral arteries in response to stimuli that release NO. Deficiency of endothelial-derived NO is believed to be the primary defect that links IR and ED.

Recently, data from epidemiological cohort studies and clinical populations have determined that OSA may contribute to the development of IR [72]. It was also reported that exposure to acute hypoxia increased glucose intolerance in healthy men and women [71]. Also showed that acute 1-day exposure to intermittent or continuous hypoxia resulted in impaired glucose tolerance, reduced insulin sensitivity, and an increased level of secretion of insulin from the pancreas [49].

In our study, we also reported a time-dependent increase in the result of the GTT, ITT, and HOMA-IR (exposure to hypoxia for up to 24 hours), which supports previous findings. Peltonen and coworkers recently reported that acute exposure to hypoxia decreases insulin sensitivity through sympathetic activation [73]. Gamboa et al. also showed that either acute exposure or continuous hypoxia can induce IR. Therefore, our conclusion is in concurrence with previous studies [71].

8. Clinical significance of the sterile inflammation and type 2 diabetes mellitus/IR

The above results implied that hypoxia-induced quantitative and qualitative changes in vWF through HMGB1-mediated activation of TLR2 and binding of SP1 to its cognate binding site on the vWF promoter. To obtain direct evidence of this transcriptional regulation by the HMGB1-TLR2-SP1-vWF-IR pathway during hypoxia and its involvement in the development of IR, we quantified the levels of HMGB1 and vWF in the plasma and those of TLR2 and SP1 in the PBMCs of diabetic and non-diabetic subjects ($n = 24$) by performing ELISA. We found that the levels of HMGB1, vWF, TLR2, and SP1 were significantly higher in diabetic subjects than in non-diabetic subjects ($p < 0.005$; **Figure 13A–D**). Next, we performed HOMA-IR in diabetic and non-diabetic subjects to confirm IR. HOMA-IR index of diabetic subjects was significantly higher than that of non-diabetic subjects (**Figure 13E**), suggesting higher IR in diabetic subjects.

9. Summary and conclusion

This research aimed to investigate hypobaric hypoxia-induced endothelial activation, inflammation, and IR. *In vivo* and *in vitro* studies were performed to accomplish the aim of the study. In brief, animals were exposed to AH at different time points and endothelial activation and IR were studied. Results showed that AH exposure upregulated the multimeric form of vWF and decreased NO production. Both vWF and NO are markers for ED. As ED and IR are interlinked in different disease and stress conditions, the parameters of glucose hemostasis were studied following AH exposure. The result showed a significant increase of GTT, ITT, and HOMA-IR in AH exposure. Our findings also suggest that AH-induced IR is mediated through inhibition of NO production. We also observed that an increased multimeric form of vWF is responsible for the inhibition of insulin-induced NO production. A glucose uptake study was conducted to demonstrate the biological relevance of AH-induced vWF upregulation & decreased NO production. The result showed that vWF inhibits glucose uptake by inhibiting NO synthesis. Therefore, these studies suggest that vWF acts as an inhibitor of NOS and impaired insulin-induced NO production.

Hypoxia induces ED by altering the endothelial-derived molecules leading to the initiation of inflammation, coagulation, and thrombogenicity. Despite the

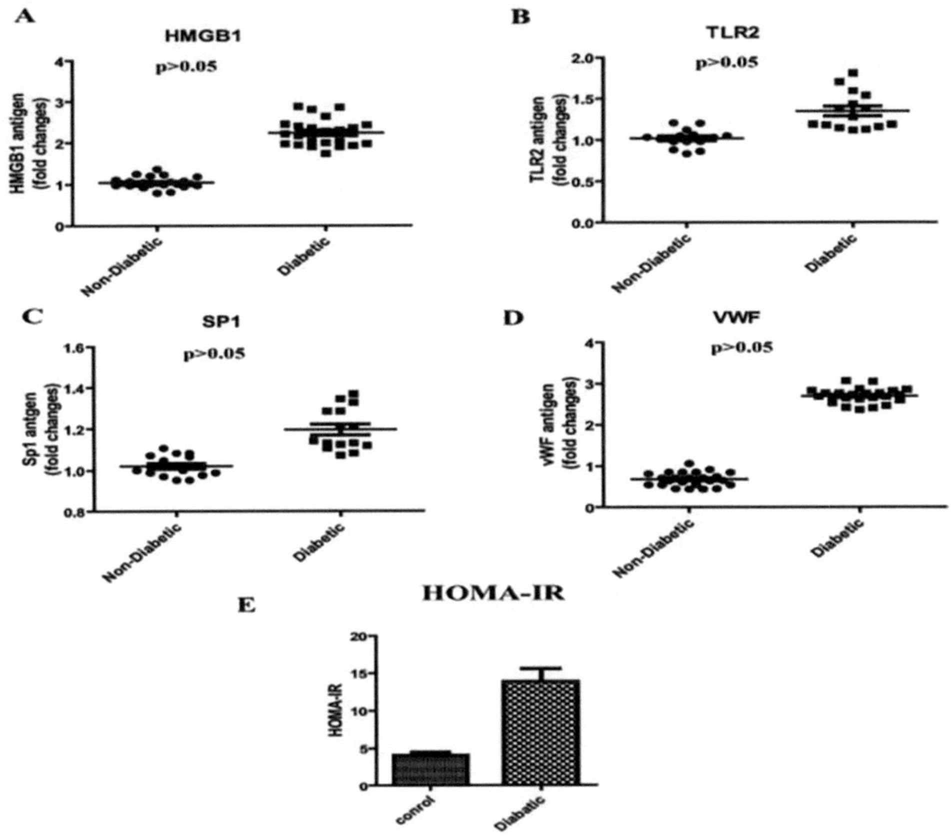

Figure 13.
*HMGB1, TLR2, SP1, and vWF in the diabetic patient sample: (A) HOMA-IR in control and diabetic patient sample (n = 24). Plasma HMGB1 (B) and vWF (E) as well as TLR2 (C) and SP1 (D) levels in PBMNC analyses by an ELISA. Data are means ± SEM of three separate experiments. The results showed a significant (*p < 0.05) difference between different time points using a one-way ANOVA.*

well-established association, we also suggest that AH-induced multimeric vWF also induced IR, but transcriptional regulation of the vWF gene during hypoxia that contributes to IR is not defined yet. Recently, it has been shown that factors released from stressed cells and tissues can function as "danger signals" and the putative ligands may activate innate immune receptors, including TLR2. The result showed TLR2 immuno-neutralization and TLR2 gene silencing significantly reduced AH-induced expression of vWF. It suggests that AH-induced vWF upregulation is regulated through TLR2. MyD88 is the most prominent adaptor protein involved in TLR2-induced vWF externalization from Weibel-Palade body. We showed an increased expression of MyD88 and phospho-SP1 following AH exposure or LTA treatment that was inhibited by TLR2 immunoneutralization or TLR2 gene silencing. Additionally, SP1 inhibitor also inhibits AH-induced vWF expression both in mRNA level as well as protein level. Our results also showed that TLR2 immunoneutralization and TLR2 gene silencing diminished the AH-induced colocalization of vWF with either MyD88 or SP1. We further demonstrated that AH-induced binding of SP1 to vWF promoter abrogated by TLR2 immunoneutralization and TLR2 gene silencing. We further observed that increased level of HMGB1 acts as an endogenous ligand for

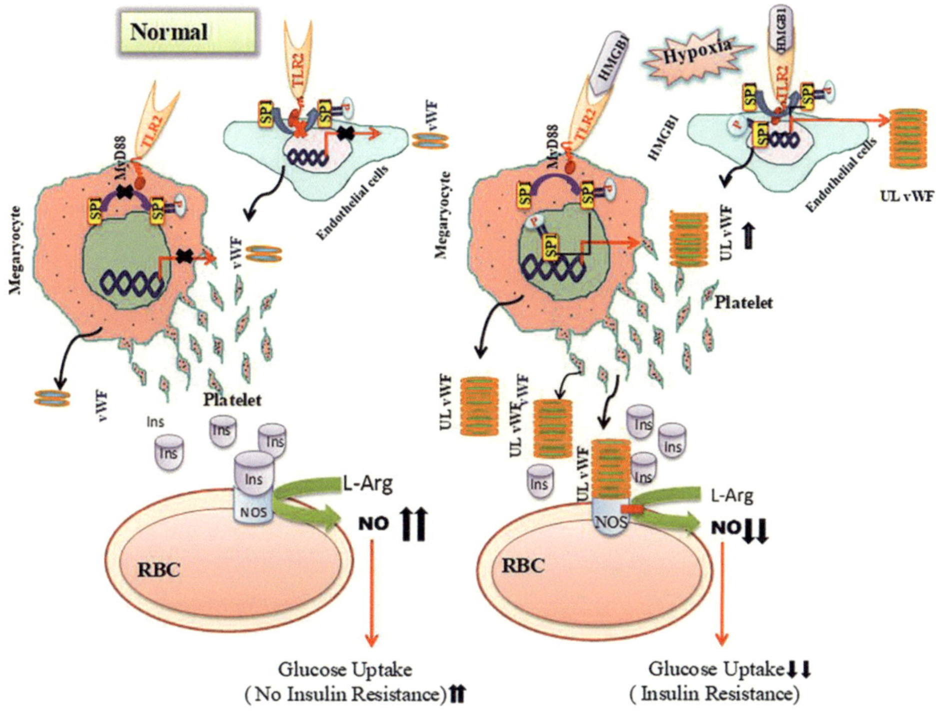

Figure 14.
Proposed model highlighting the transcriptional regulation of the vWF gene during hypoxia, which contributes to IR.

TLR2 and induces vWF upregulation during AH. From these results, we concluded that AH-induced vWF upregulation is mediated through HMGB1-TLR2-MyD88-Sp1 axis.

So, this study delineates the mechanism of inhibition of NO production and IR by vWF during hypoxia. A proposed model presented in a schematic diagram in **Figure 14**. It also explains the molecular mechanism of vWF upregulation in different stress conditions. Therefore, vWF would be potential targets for developing therapeutics in the management of stress-induced IR.

Conflict of interest

The authors assert that they do not have any conflict of interest.

Author details

Gausal A. Khan[1*], Anish Murtaja Alam Khan[2], Bandana Singh[3] and Mohammed Eid Alqahtani[4]

1 Department of Clinical Nutrition, Collage of Applied Medical Sciences, King Faisal University, Kingdom of Saudi Arabia

2 Department of Biochemistry, Hamdard Institute of Medical Science and Research (HIMSR), Jamia Hamdard, New Delhi, India

3 Department of Surgery, Boston Children's Hospital Harvard Medical School, Boston, MA, USA

4 Department of Nursing, Collage of Applied Medical Sciences, King Faisal University, Al-Ahsa, Kingdom of Saudi Arabia

*Address all correspondence to: gkhan@kfu.edu.sa; gausalk@gmail.com

References

[1] Trimarchi M, Lauritano D, Ronconi G, Caraffa A, Gallenga CE, Frydas I, et al. Mast cell cytokines in acute and chronic gingival tissue inflammation: Role of IL-33 and IL-37. International Journal of Molecular Sciences. 2022;**23**(21):1-26

[2] Chen L, Deng H, Cui H, Fang J, Zuo Z, Deng J, et al. Inflammatory responses and inflammation-associated diseases in organs. Oncotarget [Internet]. 2017;**9**(6):7204-7218. Available from: https://pubmed.ncbi.nlm.nih.gov/29467962/ [Cited 2024 May 4]

[3] Shaukat Z, Liu D, Gregory S. Sterile inflammation in drosophila. Mediators of Inflammation. 2015;**2015**:369286

[4] Asri RM, Salim E, Nainu F, Hori A, Kuraishi T. Sterile induction of innate immunity in Drosophila melanogaster. Frontiers in Bioscience-Landmark. 2019;**24**(8):1390-1400

[5] Nainu F, Salim E, Asri RM, Hori A, Kuraishi T. Neurodegenerative disorders and sterile inflammation: Lessons from a Drosophila model. Journal of Biochemistry. 2019;**166**(3):213-221

[6] Chen GY, Nuñez G. Sterile inflammation: Sensing and reacting to damage. Nature Reviews Immunology. 2010;**10**(12):826-837. Available from: https://www.nature.com/articles/nri2873

[7] Preissner KT, Fischer S, Deindl E. Extracellular RNA as a versatile DAMP and alarm signal that influences leukocyte recruitment in inflammation and infection. Frontiers in Cell and Developmental Biology. 2020;**8**:1-26. Available from: https://pubmed.ncbi.nlm.nih.gov/33392206/

[8] Bedenbender K, Schmeck BT. Endothelial ribonuclease 1 in cardiovascular and systemic inflammation. Frontiers in Cell and Development Biology. 2020;**8**:576491

[9] Chen Y, Lin J, Zhao Y, Ma X, Yi H. Toll-like receptor 3 (TLR3) regulation mechanisms and roles in antiviral innate immune responses. Journal of Zhejiang University. Science. B. 2021;**22**(8):609

[10] Son M, Diamond B, Shin JS. Editorial: The role of HMGB1 in immunity. Frontiers in Immunology. 2020;**11**:594253

[11] Zhang Y, Ehrlich SM, Zhu C, Du X. Signaling mechanisms of the platelet glycoprotein Ib-IX complex. Platelets. 2022;**33**(6):823

[12] Drakeford C, Aguila S, Roche F, Hokamp K, Fazavana J, Cervantes MP, et al. von Willebrand factor links primary hemostasis to innate immunity. Nature Communications. 2022;**13**(1):1-19. Available from: https://www.nature.com/articles/s41467-022-33796-7

[13] Chen J, Chung DW. Inflammation, von Willebrand factor, and ADAMTS13. Blood. 2018;**132**(2):141-147. DOI: 10.1182/blood-2018-02-769000

[14] Schneider MF, Fallah MA, Mess C, Obser T, Schneppenheim R, Alexander-Katz A, et al. Platelet adhesion and aggregate formation controlled by immobilised and soluble VWF. BMC Molecular and Cell Biology. 2020;**21**(1):1-13. Available from: https://bmcmolcellbiol.biomedcentral.com/articles/10.1186/s12860-020-00309-7

[15] Risser F, Urosev I, López-Morales J, Sun Y, Nash MA. Engineered molecular therapeutics targeting fibrin and the coagulation system: A biophysical

perspective. Biophysical Reviews. 2022;**14**(2):427-461. Available from: https://link.springer.com/article/10.1007/s12551-022-00950-w

[16] Choudhary S, Sharma K, Singh PK. Von Willebrand factor: A key glycoprotein involved in thrombo-inflammatory complications of COVID-19. Chemico-Biological Interactions. 2021;**348**:109657

[17] Colman, et al. Hemostasis and Thrombosis-Basic... Google Scholar. 2006. Available from: https://scholar.google.co.in/scholar?q=Colman+et+al.,%E2%80%9DHemostasis+and+Thrombosis-Basic+principles+%26+clinical+practice.%E2%80%9D&hl=en&as_sdt=0&as_vis=1&oi=scholart

[18] Schwartz BA, Fuchs B, Kannicht C, Solecka B, Kröning M. Relevance of intact Von Willebrand factor (VWF) triplet structure for VWF function. Blood. 2010;**116**(21):1425

[19] Wang W, Zhao T, Geng K, Yuan G, Chen Y, Xu Y. Smoking and the pathophysiology of peripheral artery disease. Frontiers in Cardiovascular Medicine. 2021;**8**:704106

[20] Xiang Y, Hwa J. Regulation of VWF expression, and secretion in health and disease. Current Opinion in Hematology. 2016;**23**(3):288

[21] Geggel RL, Carvalho ACA, Hoyer LW, Reid LM. von Willebrand factor abnormalities in primary pulmonary hypertension. The American Review of Respiratory Disease. 1987;**135**(2):294-299. Available from: https://pubmed.ncbi.nlm.nih.gov/3101558/

[22] Anyanwagu U, Donnelly R, Idris I. The relationship between urinary albumin excretion, cardiovascular outcomes and total mortality among a large cohort of insulin-treated patients with type 2 diabetes in routine primary care practices. Nephrology, Dialysis, Transplantation. 2020;**35**(3):471-477. Available from: https://pubmed.ncbi.nlm.nih.gov/30169825/

[23] van Paridon PCS, Panova-Noeva M, van Oerle R, Schulz A, Prochaska JH, Arnold N, et al. Lower levels of vWF are associated with lower risk of cardiovascular disease. Research and Practice in Thrombosis and Haemostasis. 2022;**6**(7):4-26

[24] Manz XD, Bogaard HJ, Aman J. Regulation of VWF (Von Willebrand factor) in inflammatory thrombosis. Arteriosclerosis, Thrombosis, and Vascular Biology. 2022;**42**(11):1307-1320. Available from: https://www.ahajournals.org/doi/abs/10.1161/ATVBAHA.122.318179

[25] Frankel DS, Meigs JB, Massaro JM. Von Willebrand factor, type 2 diabetes mellitus, and risk of cardiovascular disease: The Framingham offspring study. Journal of Vascular Surgery. 2009;**50**(1):235. Available from: http://www.jvascsurg.org/article/S0741521409011653/fulltext

[26] Davies MG, Hagen PO. The vascular endothelium. A new horizon. Annals of Surgery. 1993;**218**(5):593-609. Available from: https://pubmed.ncbi.nlm.nih.gov/8239773/

[27] Atiq F, Meijer K, Eikenboom J, Fijnvandraat K, Mauser-Bunschoten EP, van Galen KPM, et al. Comorbidities associated with higher von Willebrand factor (VWF) levels may explain the age-related increase of VWF in von Willebrand disease. British Journal of Haematology. 2018;**182**(1):93-105. Available from: https://onlinelibrary.wiley.com/doi/full/10.1111/bjh.15277

[28] Herrick AL. Pathogenesis of Raynaud's phenomenon. Rheumatology. 2005;**44**(5):587-596. DOI: 10.1093/rheumatology/keh552

[29] Patnaik E, Lyons M, Tran K, Pattanaik D. Endothelial dysfunction in systemic sclerosis. International Journal of Molecular Sciences. 2023;**24**(18):7-23

[30] Xia C, Braunstein Z, Toomey AC, Zhong J, Rao X. S100 proteins as an important regulator of macrophage inflammation. Frontiers in Immunology. 2018;**8**:316508

[31] Singh P, Ali SA, Kalyuzhny E, Singh P, Ali SA. Multifunctional role of S100 protein family in the immune system: An update. Cells. 2022;**11**(15):2274. Available from: https://www.mdpi.com/2073-4409/11/15/2274/htm

[32] Riuzzi F, Beccafico S, Sagheddu R, Chiappalupi S, Giambanco I, Bereshchenko O, et al. Levels of S100B protein drive the reparative process in acute muscle injury and muscular dystrophy. Scientific Reports. 2017;7(1):1-16. Available from: https://www.nature.com/articles/s41598-017-12880-9

[33] Moysa A, Steczkiewicz K, Niedzialek D, Hammerschmid D, Zhukova L, Sobott F, et al. A model of full-length RAGE in complex with S100B. Structure. 2021;**29**(9):989-1002.e6. Available from: https://pubmed.ncbi.nlm.nih.gov/33887170/

[34] Roche M, Michetti F, Di SG, Clementi ME, Valeriani F, Mandarano M, et al. The multifaceted S100B protein: A role in obesity and diabetes? International Journal of Molecular Sciences. 2024;**25**(2):776. Available from: https://www.mdpi.com/1422-0067/25/2/776/htm

[35] Van EW, Jansen MAA, Ludwig IS, Leufkens P, Goes C, VanLaar JM, et al. Heat shock proteins can be surrogate autoantigens for induction of antigen specific therapeutic tolerance in rheumatoid arthritis. Frontiers in Immunology. 2019;**10**:439708

[36] Tukaj S, Mantej J, Sobala M, Potrykus K, Sitko K. Autologous extracellular Hsp70 exerts a dual role in rheumatoid arthritis. Cell Stress & Chaperones. 2020;**25**(6):1105

[37] Wilson JW, Shakir D, Batie M, Frost M, Rocha S. Oxygen-sensing mechanisms in cells. The FEBS Journal. 2020;**287**(18):3888-3906. Available from: https://onlinelibrary.wiley.com/doi/full/10.1111/febs.15374

[38] Fuhrmann DC, Brüne B. Mitochondrial composition and function under the control of hypoxia. Redox Biology. 2017;**12**:208

[39] Kahan R, Cray PL, Abraham N, Gao Q, Hartwig MG, Pollara JJ, et al. Sterile inflammation in liver transplantation. Frontiers in Medicine (Lausanne). 2023;**10**:10-26. Available from: https://pubmed.ncbi.nlm.nih.gov/37636574/

[40] Chen GY, Nuñez G. Sterile inflammation: Sensing and reacting to damage. Nature Reviews Immunology. 2010;**10**(12):826-837. Available from: https://www.nature.com/articles/nri2873

[41] Hally K, Fauteux-Daniel S, Hamzeh-Cognasse H, Larsen P, Cognasse F. Revisiting platelets and toll-like receptors (TLRs): At the interface of vascular immunity and thrombosis. International Journal of Molecular Sciences. 2020;**21**(17):6150. Available from: https://www.mdpi.com/1422-0067/21/17/6150/htm

[42] Blair P, Rex S, Vitseva O, Beaulieu L, Tanriverdi K, Chakrabarti S,

et al. Stimulation of toll-like receptor 2 in human platelets induces a thromboinflammatory response through activation of phosphoinositide 3-kinase. Circulation Research. 2009;**104**(3):346-354. Available from: https://pubmed.ncbi.nlm.nih.gov/19106411/

[43] Jin M, Fang J, Wang JJ, Shao X, Xu S-W, Liu P-Q, et al. Regulation of toll-like receptor (TLR) signaling pathways in atherosclerosis: From mechanisms to targeted therapeutics. Acta Pharmacologica Sinica. 2023;**44**(12):2358-2375. Available from: https://www.nature.com/articles/s41401-023-01123-5

[44] Vadapalli S, Surekha Rani H, Sastry BKS, Nallari P. Endothelin-1 and endothelial nitric oxide polymorphisms in idiopathic pulmonary arterial hypertension. International Journal of Molecular Epidemiology and Genetics. 2010;**1**(3):208

[45] Yang J, Jia Z, Song X, Shi J, Wang X, Zhao X, et al. Proteomic and clinical biomarkers for acute mountain sickness in a longitudinal cohort. Communications Biology. 2022;**5**(1):11-12

[46] Kubisz P, Stančiaková L, Staško J, Galajda P, Mokáň M. Endothelial and platelet markers in diabetes mellitus type 2. World Journal of Diabetes. 2015;**6**(3):423

[47] Morganti A, Marana I, Airoldi F, Alberti C, Nador B, Palatresi S. Plasma endothelin levels: A meaningless number? Journal of Cardiovascular Pharmacology. 2000;**4**(2). Available from: https://journals.lww.com/cardiovascularpharm/fulltext/2000/00002/plasma_endothelin_levels__a_meaningless_number_.6.aspx

[48] Baaten CCFMJ, Vondenhoff S, Noels H. Endothelial cell dysfunction and increased cardiovascular risk in patients with chronic kidney disease. Circulation Research. 2023;**132**(8):970-992. Available from: https://www.ahajournals.org/doi/abs/10.1161/CIRCRESAHA.123.321752

[49] van Hulten V, van Meijel RLJ, Goossens GH. The impact of hypoxia exposure on glucose homeostasis in metabolically compromised humans: A systematic review. Reviews in Endocrine & Metabolic Disorders. 2021;**22**(2):471-483. Available from: https://link.springer.com/article/10.1007/s11154-021-09654-0

[50] Pramsohler S, Burtscher M, Rausch L, Netzer NC. Weight loss and fat metabolism during multi-day high-altitude sojourns: A hypothesis based on adipocyte signaling. Life. 2022;**12**(4):545. Available from: https://www.mdpi.com/2075-1729/12/4/545/htm

[51] Wagner PD. Operation Everest II. High Altitude Medicine & Biology. 2010;**11**(2):111

[52] Koh HCE, van Vliet S, Cao C, Patterson BW, Reeds DN, Laforest R, et al. Effect of obstructive sleep apnea on glucose metabolism. European Journal of Endocrinology. 2022;**186**(4):457-467. Available from: https://pubmed.ncbi.nlm.nih.gov/35118996/

[53] Jaitovich A, Jourd'heuil D. A brief overview of nitric oxide and reactive oxygen species signaling in hypoxia-induced pulmonary hypertension. Advances in Experimental Medicine and Biology. 2017;**967**:71

[54] Singh B, Biswas I, Garg I, Sugadev R, Singh AK, Dey S, et al. von Willebrand factor antagonizes nitric oxide synthase to promote insulin resistance during hypoxia. Biochemistry. 2014;**53**(1):115-126. DOI: 10.1021/bi401061e

[55] Bahadoran Z, Mirmiran P, Kashfi K, Ghasemi A. Vascular nitric

oxide resistance in type 2 diabetes. Cell Death & Disease. 2023;**14**(7):1-14. Available from: https://www.nature.com/articles/s41419-023-05935-5

[56] Frankel DS, Meigs JB, Massaro JM, Wilson PWF, O'Donnell CJ, D'Agostino RB, et al. Von Willebrand factor, type 2 diabetes and risk of cardiovascular disease: The Framingham offspring study. Circulation. 2008;**118**(24):2533

[57] Waterhouse A, Bertoni M, Bienert S, Studer G, Tauriello G, Gumienny R, et al. SWISS-MODEL: Homology modelling of protein structures and complexes. Nucleic Acids Research. 2018;**46**(W1):W296-W303. DOI: 10.1093/nar/gky427

[58] Guex N, Peitsch MC. SWISS-MODEL and the Swiss-Pdb viewer: An environment for comparative protein modeling. Electrophoresis. 1997;**18**(15):2714-2723. Available from: https://onlinelibrary.wiley.com/doi/full/10.1002/elps.1150181505

[59] Guex N, Peitsch MC, Schwede T. Automated comparative protein structure modeling with SWISS-MODEL and Swiss-PdbViewer: A historical perspective. Electrophoresis. 2009;**30**(Suppl 1(SUPPL. 1)). Available from: https://pubmed.ncbi.nlm.nih.gov/19517507/

[60] Holdsworth G, Roberts SJ, Ke HZ. Novel actions of sclerostin on bone. Journal of Molecular Endocrinology. 2019;**62**(2):R167-R185. Available from: https://jme.bioscientifica.com/view/journals/jme/62/2/JME-18-0176.xml

[61] Menting JG, Whittaker J, Margetts MB, Whittaker LJ, Kong GKW, Smith BJ, et al. How insulin engages its primary binding site on the insulin receptor. Nature. 2013;**493**(7431):241-245. Available from: https://www.nature.com/articles/nature11781

[62] Uchikawa E, Choi E, Shang G, Yu H, Xiao-Chen B. Activation mechanism of the insulin receptor revealed by cryo-EM structure of the fully liganded receptor-ligand complex. eLife. 2019;**8**:21-22

[63] Arnett DK, Blumenthal RS, Albert M, Buroker AB, et al. Writing committee members circulation. Circulation. ACC/AHA Guideline on the Primary Prevention of Cardiovascular Disease: A Report of the American College of Cardiology/American Heart Association Task Force on Clinical Practice Guidelines. 2019;**140**:596-646. Available from: http://ahajournals.org

[64] Wittwer J, Bradley D. Clusterin and its role in insulin resistance and the Cardiometabolic syndrome. Frontiers in Immunology. 2021;**12**:612496

[65] Badran M, Golbidi S, Ayas N, Laher I. Nitric oxide bioavailability in obstructive sleep apnea: Interplay of asymmetric dimethylarginine and free radicals. Sleep Disorders. 2015;**2015**:1-10

[66] Gheibi S, Ghasemi A. Insulin secretion: The nitric oxide controversy. EXCLI Journal. 2020;**19**:1227

[67] Nakhaei-Nejad M, Farhan M, Mojiri A, Jabbari H, Murray AG, Jahroudi N. Regulation of von Willebrand factor gene in endothelial cells that are programmed to pluripotency and differentiated Back to endothelial cells. Stem Cells. 2019;**37**(4):22-23. Available from: https://pubmed.ncbi.nlm.nih.gov/30682218/

[68] Hong YH, Betik AC, Mcconell GK. Role of nitric oxide in skeletal muscle glucose uptake during exercise. Experimental Physiology.

2014;**99**(12):1569-1573. Available from: https://onlinelibrary.wiley.com/doi/full/10.1113/expphysiol.2014.079202

[69] Chakraborty K, Khan GA, Banerjee P, Ray U, Sinha AK. Inhibition of human blood platelet aggregation and the stimulation of nitric oxide synthesis by aspirin. Platelets. 2003;**14**(7-8):421-427. Available from: https://www.tandfonline.com/doi/abs/10.1080/09537103200 0158763

[70] Merry TL, McConell GK. Skeletal muscle glucose uptake during exercise: A focus on reactive oxygen species and nitric oxide signaling. IUBMB Life. 2009;**61**(5):479-484. Available from: https://pubmed.ncbi.nlm.nih.gov/19391163/

[71] Song K, Zhang Y, Ga Q, Bai Z, Ge RL. Increased insulin sensitivity by high-altitude hypoxia in mice with high-fat diet-induced obesity is associated with activated AMPK signaling and subsequently enhanced mitochondrial biogenesis in skeletal muscles. Obesity Facts. 2020;**13**(5):455

[72] Punjabi NM, Shahar E, Redline S, Gottlieb DJ, Givelber R, Resnick HE. Sleep-disordered breathing, glucose intolerance, and insulin resistance: The Sleep Heart Health Study. American Journal of Epidemiology. 2004;**160**(6):521-530. Available from: https://pubmed.ncbi.nlm.nih.gov/15353412/

[73] Poulain L, Mathieu H, Thomas A, Borel AL, Remy C, Levy P, et al. Intermittent hypoxia-induced insulin resistance is associated with alterations in white fat distribution. Scientific Reports. 2017;**7**(1):1-9. Available from: https://www.nature.com/articles/s41598-017-11782-0

Chapter 8

Lifestyle Interventions to Manage Insulin Resistance

Olorunfemi Oyewole Babalola, Paul Olamide Ottu, Ebenezer Akinnusi, Precious Olayinka Aturamu and Opeyemi Iwaloye

Abstract

This chapter will discuss chronic stress, which is the final phase of the comprehensive method. Both mindfulness and meditation have demonstrated the potential as therapeutic practices in their respective fields of study. Those individuals and healthcare professionals who are interested in addressing insulin sensitivity and improving metabolic health in a holistic manner will find the insights that are presented in this chapter to be extremely beneficial. In this chapter, a paradigm shift that takes into account all aspects of lifestyle is advocated for.

Keywords: insulin sensitivity, chronic stress, mindfulness, meditation, holistic health

1. Introduction

In glucose metabolism, insulin is crucial. After eating carbohydrates, the body breaks them down into glucose, which enters the bloodstream. Insulin, produced by the pancreas, helps cells absorb glucose to regulate blood sugar. Insulin resistance can reduce cell response to this hormone. Thus, insulin resistance diminishes cell sensitivity to insulin, which regulates glucose absorption. This complicated phenomena influence system and cell homeostasis simultaneously. Pancreatic insulin regulates glucose metabolism and helps cells absorb glucose by attaching to the cell surface receptors [1]. This aids glucose absorption by liver, muscle, and fat cells. In insulin resistance, this signaling system is disrupted, reducing cell glucose uptake and utilization.

Insulin resistance affects more than glucose metabolism. Insulin resistance causes chronic hyperglycemia, endothelial dysfunction, oxidative stress, and inflammation, which cause cardiovascular diseases [2]. Insulin resistance and β-cell dysfunction are common observations in type 2 diabetes mellitus (T2DM). Resistance increases strain on pancreatic β-cells, leading to fatigue and decreased insulin output. The vicious cycle of β-cell dysfunction and insulin resistance worsens T2DM [3]. Lipid metabolic dysregulation—low dense LDL particles, low HDL-C, and high triglycerides—is also caused by insulin resistance. Additionally, lipid abnormalities cause cardiovascular disease-related atherosclerosis [4].

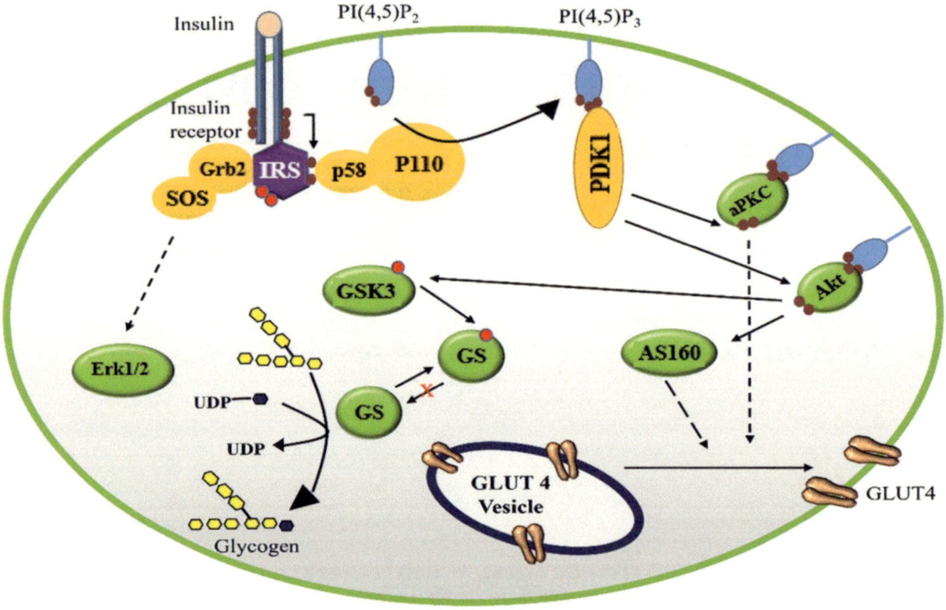

Figure 1.
Diagram showing insulin resistance's defective signaling pathway: Disruptions in insulin receptor substrate 1 signaling affect glucose transport. Under normal physiological settings, insulin binds to cell surface receptors to start the insulin signaling cascade in skeletal muscle and adipose tissue. IRS-1 phosphorylation stimulates insulin receptor and PPIK-3 kinase. Protein kinase B/Akt phosphorylates AS160 and activates Rab proteins to transfer GLUT4 vesicles to the cell membrane when PI3K is activated. GLUT4 transfers glucose within the cell for metabolism or storage from the cell surface.

Insulin resistance is an important public health issue today. Genetic, environmental, and modern sedentary lifestyle factors promote insulin resistance. Inactivity and sedentary habits cause obesity and metabolic disorders. Skeletal muscle glucose transport and use increase insulin resistance [4]. Overeating processed foods, high-fat diets, and calories can also develop insulin resistance [5]. Diets heavy in saturated fat and carbs produce obesity and other metabolic issues that worsen insulin resistance. Preventing insulin resistance health issues requires preventive actions. Insulin resistance is a prelude to significant health issues, thus early intervention reduces risk and improves results (**Figure 1**).

2. Influences of dietary choices on insulin response

Treatment of metabolic syndrome problems, including insulin resistance, involves diet and lifestyle changes. This technique aims to reduce body weight, improve glycemic control, and reduce the risk of cardiovascular disease and other consequences, which account for 80% of diabetes-related fatalities [6]. For insulin resistance hyperglycemia, contemporary diets recommend complex carbohydrates or starches over simple carbs and sweets. This technique ignores metabolic evidence showing certain starchy meals, such as baked potatoes and white bread, may increase glycemic responses and believes that simple sugars are absorbed and digested quicker, resulting in a faster postprandial glucose response [7]. Generalizations concerning carbohydrate consumption and insulin resistance, obesity, and diabetes have arisen from conceptual uncertainty about dietary carbs and the widespread use of low-carb diets for weight reduction.

Excess sugar consumption directly and indirectly accelerates insulin resistance. Overeating sugar generates a positive energy balance, which increases body weight and fat. Additionally, it indirectly induces insulin resistance and glucose dysregulation. Fructose raises ghrelin, the hunger hormone, and lowers hypothalamic malonyl-CoA [8], which increases appetite, weight, and insulin sensitivity. Inflammation and hepatic fat buildup from these carbohydrates may cause insulin resistance. Fructose, a lipogenic sugar, is primarily metabolized in the liver and seldom reaches the circulation [9]. GLUT2 processes fructose into fructose-1-phosphate, dihydroxyacetone phosphate, and glyceraldehyde 3-phosphate, which increases *de novo* lipogenesis [10]. Fructose may impair hepatic fatty acid oxidation by inducing mitochondrial oxidative stress via uric acid [11]. In Havel's human experiments, fructose-sweetened drinks enhanced lipogenesis, dyslipidemia, and circulating uric acid while lowering insulin sensitivity and fatty acid oxidation. These changes in fructose and glucose's hepatic metabolism, including how they enter the glycolytic pathway and what happens to their intermediary metabolites, may explain these effects [8, 10].

Dietary fat strongly predicts insulin resistance in humans and animals. In humans, total fat consumption substantially elevates HbA1c, 2-hour post-load glucose, and fasting insulin. A 40 g/d increase in dietary fat increases T2DM risk 3.4-fold [8]. Saturated and unsaturated lipids affect insulin resistance differently. Polyunsaturated fat improves insulin sensitivity and glucose tolerance, while saturated fat is linked to insulin resistance and T2DM in most epidemiologic and clinical investigations [8]. The advantages of a monounsaturated fatty acid-rich diet decrease when total fat consumption surpasses 38% [12]. Variable fatty acid carbon chain lengths affect insulin sensitivity. Long-chain fatty acids (LCFAs, >C16) make up most western diet fats and are linked to glucose homeostasis and insulin resistance [13]. Compared to LCFAs with equivalent calories, medium-chain fatty acids (MCFAs, C8–C12) reduce obesity and enhance insulin action by increasing energy expenditure and fatty acid oxidation [8]. Gut microbiomes ferment indigestible food into C2–C6 SCFAs. SCFAs improve liver, skeletal muscle, and adipose tissue insulin sensitivity [14]. Nutritional fat intake and quality are critical to T2DM.

Overweight increases metabolic syndrome and insulin resistance risk. Overeating and metabolically active abdominal adipose tissue increase the non-esterified fatty acid transport to the liver, which may impair insulin extraction, glucose oxidation, and insulin secretion. T2DM intervention studies show that weight reduction decreases fasting hyperglycemia, boosts non-oxidative glucose metabolism, and improves insulin sensitivity [15]. Unbalanced energy intake and expenditure cause obesity. Calorie intake from sedentary lifestyles and high-fat diets causes overweight. High-fat, high-energy diets may cause insulin resistance, glucose intolerance, obesity, cardiovascular disease, and metabolic syndrome [16]. Several clinical researches support this notion. Saturated fat may increase metabolic problems, although monounsaturated fat may improve lipids. Epidemiological research suggests trans-fatty acids increase T2DM and insulin resistance [17]. Saturated and certain monounsaturated fats cause insulin resistance but not polyunsaturated or omega-3 s [17]. Dietary fat affects insulin sensitivity regardless of weight and increases T2DM risk [15]. Numerous research on people and animals have connected reduced insulin sensitivity to dietary fat quality, perhaps owing to cell membrane fatty acid composition changes [18]. Understanding macronutrient satiation and energy overconsumption is crucial. Due to their great palatability, high-fat meals may induce passive overconsumption [17]. Even though both dietary energy intake and macronutrient quality contribute to obesity and insulin resistance, dietitians and other health professionals must continue to challenge the quantity and quality of macronutrients in food and diet composition to develop novel ways to reduce metabolic syndrome-related insulin resistance.

2.1 Dietary strategies for improving insulin sensitivity

In an effort to increase insulin sensitivity, several dietary approaches have been used throughout time, such as whole food-based diets. Plant-based foods in their whole, minimally processed, unprocessed form make up these diets. They include a variety of foods such legumes, fruits, vegetables, whole grains, seeds, nuts, and beans, as well as small amounts of healthy fats. When it comes to the ratio of nutrients to calories, whole foods have a greater content of the important nutrients than processed meals. They serve as excellent sources of dietary fiber, antioxidants, and phytochemicals and provide essential vitamins, minerals, fiber, and phytonutrients necessary for metabolic health.

Diets centered on whole foods can maintain a healthy gut microbiota, balance macronutrient consumption, improve heart health, help control weight, and lower insulin resistance [19]. For example, increasing insulin sensitivity and controlling blood sugar levels may be achieved by including whole grains, veggies, and legumes in one's diet. Blood sugar spikes are avoided by energy-restricted diets that include a balanced mix of proteins, lipids, and carbs. Eating complex carbs that have a low GI helps to reduce blood sugar spikes and promote constant glucose release. Furthermore, including good fats—like omega-3 fatty acids—and keeping protein consumption modest promote muscle health without producing an excessive amount of insulin. Reducing the consumption of added sugars, maintaining regular meal timings, staying hydrated, and including turmeric and cinnamon into meals are other successful dietary methods to improve insulin sensitivity [20, 21].

2.2 Benefits of a whole-foods-based diet in managing insulin resistance

A substantial body of literature has given reports that revealed the profound impact of whole foods based diet such as whole grain, fruits, vegetables, and legumes on insulin resistance and broader metabolic health. Literature consistently supports the notion that whole foods exert substantial and multifaceted benefits on insulin sensitivity. Arabzadega et al. research outcomes revealed that the consumption of the whole grains, characterized by higher fiber content and a lower glycemic index modulates insulin sensitivity [22]. Wallace et al. demonstrated that the antioxidants and fiber present in fruits exhibited a significant improvement on glucose metabolism, positioning fruits as a protective factor against insulin resistance [23]. Furthermore, it has been shown in the previous research that consuming more veggies is linked to lower insulin levels and higher insulin sensitivity. This result bolsters the notion that a broad range of vegetables should be included in dietary guidelines [24]. Legumes are a desired alternative for those trying to cure insulin resistance since their consumption has been linked to benefits in glycemic control and insulin sensitivity. Legumes like beans, lentils, and peas are regarded as important nutritional sources that are required to keep the metabolism functioning properly. Eating a diet high in fruits, vegetables, whole grains, and legumes is linked to synergistic benefits since it effectively improves insulin sensitivity and lowers the risk factors linked to hypertension [25].

2.3 Mechanisms: unraveling the complex biology of improved insulin sensitivity through whole-food-based diets

Many studies have been conducted on the intricate biochemical mechanisms via which a diet high in whole foods increases insulin sensitivity. Previous research has shown the multifaceted impact of diet on metabolic health. The high fiber content of whole meals improves sensitivity to insulin. Fiber lowers the postprandial hyperglycemia spikes by slowing the absorption of glucose. Fiber enhances postprandial glucose regulation and insulin sensitivity, according to research by Fujii et al. [26]. Whole meals include phytochemicals and antioxidants that increase insulin sensitivity. Polyphenols found in fruits and vegetables improve insulin signaling and lessen oxidative damage. Whole meals alter gut flora and encourage the cooperation of host and bacteria. The diverse gut flora that is produced by fruits, vegetables, and whole grains has an impact on metabolic signaling and insulin sensitivity [27]. Hormones that control glucose homeostasis, such as insulin and glucagon, are impacted by whole meals. Whole food-based diets enhance insulin sensitivity and glucose metabolism [28].

Bioactive compounds included in whole foods regulate insulin sensitivity and energy balance via enhancing mitochondrial activity. Bioactive compounds included in fruits and vegetables may influence the expression of genes related to glucose metabolism and insulin signaling via epigenetic mechanisms, according to Čí et al. [29, 30]. The control of epigenetics implies that dietary modifications might impact metabolic health in the long run. Whole food diets with immune-modulating properties have been shown to lessen metabolic dysfunction. Whole fruits and vegetables improve insulin sensitivity and reduce inflammatory markers [30, 31]. These studies show that whole foods-based diets are helpful in enhancing insulin sensitivity due to a complex combination of metabolic processes, mitochondrial function, fiber, antioxidants, gut flora, omega-3 fatty acids, hormone control, and inflammatory modulation. Customized dietary recommendations to address insulin resistance are made possible by these interconnected pathways, which provide a holistic understanding of how nutrition influences metabolic health.

3. Physical activity, exercise, and insulin sensitivity

It is now well acknowledged that engaging in consistent physical activity is a beneficial treatment approach that may enhance insulin action in skeletal muscle in those who are thought to be insulin-resistant. It has been shown that exercise training dramatically lowers the likelihood of insulin resistance in those who are more likely to develop T2DM [32]. By increasing these people's insulin activity and glucose tolerance, this is achieved.

3.1 Aerobic and resistance training for insulin sensitivity

For individuals with Type 2 Diabetes Mellitus (T2DM), it is advisable to engage in both resistance and aerobic exercises. The treatment for T2DM involves aerobic exercise training [33]. Exercise lowers metabolic risk factors for cardiovascular disease, improves insulin sensitivity, and manages diabetes. Enhancing insulin response to glucose and glucose tolerance via endurance exercise may help reduce blood sugar. Adult obesity increases in insulin sensitivity with brief training are comparable [34].

Resistance training is known to have a far smaller impact on some of these outcomes than aerobic training, such as glycogen synthase activity. Resistance training had little effect on pro-inflammatory markers, according to other research [35]. However, reductions in adipose mass [36] have an impact on some inflammation markers, including as IL-6 and resistin, which can be increased or stimulated by resistance training. Insulin resistance and glycemic control may both be improved by resistance training and muscle building exercise regimens. Moreover, it has been shown that combining resistance and aerobic exercise improves the function of endothelial vasodilators, which may raise blood flow and glucose absorption into active muscle beds. Thus, it has been shown that, perhaps via different mechanisms, strength training and aerobic exercise are beneficial for people with T2DM [37]. Improvements in psychosocial factors and/or β-adrenergic receptor pathways may partially mediate the lowering of serum inflammatory cytokines, such as IL-18, CRP, and IL-6, in older persons, but aerobic exercise intervention does not [38]. Exercise's proposed methods for reducing inflammation include the cholinergic anti-inflammatory pathway, muscle-released interleukin-6 inhibiting tumor necrosis factor-α, and decreased proportion of body fat and macrophage buildup in adipose tissue. Reduced levels of circulating TNF-α and IL-6 may be linked to the positive effects of exercise, which could lead to reduced endothelial dysfunction and insulin resistance [39]. An increase in adiponectin levels and a decrease in C-reactive protein were observed during a 12-week swimming program conducted three times a week, which was linked to improved assessments of chronic inflammatory markers. Changes in these inflammatory mediators seemed to be connected to improvements in insulin sensitivity brought on by swimming exercise. Along with a decrease in visceral adipose tissue and waist circumference, it also led to a significant drop in circulating IL-6 in lean, obese, and T2DM participants who followed an exercise program without losing weight [40].

Both aerobic and resistance physical activity can alter body composition, substrate metabolism, signaling pathways, and organ function, which ultimately increases insulin sensitivity and improves metabolic regulation in individuals with prediabetes. Although many pathways that increase insulin sensitivity are common to both aerobic and resistance training, each modality offers unique and complimentary effects [41]. The greatest changes as a result of resistance training occur through changes in muscle strength and mass, although improvements in insulin sensitivity via increased GLUT4 expression can also occur. The evidence for aerobic physical activity-related changes on whole-body insulin sensitivity and consequent cardiometabolic protection is more widespread and involves multiple tissues and organs [42].

3.2 The role of regular physical activity in maintaining insulin sensitivity

The purpose of physical exercise is to maintain or improve one's physical condition through planned, repetitive movements. Highly trained athletes are able to perform well because exercise training alters their metabolism. Furthermore, adaptations to exercise dramatically change resting metabolism. Numerous tactics have the potential to enhance glucose excretion and insulin sensitivity. Studies that compare trained and untrained individuals show the extent of this effect, even if they cannot completely rule out population differences resulting from natural selection. The insulin response, baseline insulin level, and insulin levels after continuous glucose infusion were all 50% lower in trained subjects than in matching untrained subjects [43]. The euglycemic clamp demonstrated that individuals with training had either enhanced or equal [43] insulin responsiveness, as well as greater insulin sensitivity (submaximal insulin stimulation).

Exercises involving resistance and aerobics must be distinguished. An hour of moderate-intensity aerobic exercise lowers body fat and enhances oxygen utilization and delivery in the heart and skeletal muscle [44, 45]. Aerobic exercises include riding a bike, running, and jumping rope. On the other hand, resistance training, which repeats weight or free weight loads, is a brief strength training regimen that builds lean body mass [44, 45]. Both forms of exercise can occasionally help young people's obesity-related health. Rope jumping has been demonstrated in prehypertensive girls to improve lean body mass and decrease abdominal obesity [46]. Due to the fact that exercise influences insulin resistance, scientists started contrasting how various forms of exercise affected these variables. Van der Heijden et al. found that a 12-week aerobic training program decreased insulin resistance and the deposition of hepatic and visceral fat in obese children. During aerobic exercise, muscle cells take up more glucose, which increases glucose oxidation [47]. Lowering insulin levels reduces insulin resistance, and this mechanism controls the release of glucose and insulin [48, 49]. Children who received 16 weeks of resistance training had reduced fasting insulin levels and increased insulin sensitivity, according to studies by Refs [50, 51]. Resistance training raises skeletal muscle mass, which raises metabolic "reserve" for glucose disposal, and muscle contractions, which temporarily boost glucose uptake. These two factors together improve insulin sensitivity. Aerobic + resistance training was shown to reduce fasting insulin levels, increase insulin resistance, and improve glucose elimination in multiple investigations [52, 53]. Eight weeks of combined training increased insulin sensitivity by 22.2%, according to Refs. [54].

3.3 Effects of exercise on insulin resistance: molecular perspective

Numerous biological processes allow exercise to increase insulin sensitivity. GLUT-4, the glucose transporter, is activated by exercise and aids in the absorption of glucose by skeletal muscle in the absence of insulin. Rats that exercise for 8 weeks show a 100-fold increase in GLUT-4 translocation and receptor activation [55]. Human muscle biopsy samples exhibited GLUT-4 translocation to the plasma membrane during exercise [56]. Numerous studies have shown the impact of physical exercise on the transcription factor PPAR γ co-activator 1a (PGC-1α) and its downstream genes [57]. Phenotypic fatty acid oxidation genes are enhanced and skeletal muscle lipid intake is limited when PGC-1α activates PPARγ. Mitochondrial biogenesis is one of the processes in which PGC-1α is involved. Even while insulin resistance leads to mitochondrial dysfunction, exercise enhances the size, quantity, oxidative capacity, and biogenesis of mitochondria [58]. Exercise improves mitochondrial activity, modifies the makeup of adipokines, and reduces inflammatory indicators after oxidative damage. Furthermore, via decreasing IRS-1, GLUT-4, and PGC-1α and increasing Ser/Thr phosphorylation kinase, TNF-α and IL-6 also contribute to increased insulin resistance [59].

3.4 Incorporating regular physical activity into daily life

Regardless of the methods used to assess insulin sensitivity/glycemic control, a lifestyle incorporating regular physical activity has been identified as a key factor for maintaining and improving many aspects of health, including insulin sensitivity [60]. In this context, the term physical activity covers all forms of muscular movement, including that associated with strenuous physical work, active transport (walking and cycling), household tasks (cleaning and gardening), incidental physical activity which occurs when undertaking other tasks, sport, and other active leisure pursuits have the specific intent of affecting an aspect of health [61].

Several studies have identified an association between regular physical activity and/or aerobic fitness, one of such study explained that exercise interventions have an ameliorative effect or in some cases, lead to complete reversal of insulin resistance thereby, reducing the risk of T2D by ~9% [62]. Physical activity has both immediate (acute) and longer-term effects on insulin sensitivity. The immediate effects are the direct result of a single exercise bout and may be evident during and/or for up to 72 hours post-exercise [63]. If repeated regularly these bouts produce additional long-term chronic improvements to insulin sensitivity, thereby providing superior baseline glycemic control compared with that typically seen in less active individuals [60]. In this healthy, physically active, "trained" condition, the effects of individual exercise bouts may then produce further acute responses from this already elevated insulin sensitivity state and thereby promote optimal insulin sensitivity and glycemic control.

3.5 Practical tips for incorporating exercise into our routine

As such, individuals should be slowly introduced to both aerobic and resistance exercises to avoid injury and dropout as a result of being overwhelmed. Patients should be made aware that resistance exercise improves health risks and quality of life, but it takes time and effort to achieve its advantages, which include decreased body fat and increased muscle mass. It is important to prioritize physical activity as part of a lifestyle change rather than just structured exercise. Participants may choose more energy-dense lifestyles such as athletics, dance, gaming, and daily living. There are other options, including bicycling instead of driving or using the stairs instead of the elevator. Patients with metabolic dysfunction must exercise often. Bouts of physical activity should be performed with a high frequency on most, if not all, days of the week [64], with 72 hours between workouts. This allows individuals to optimize the transient effects of physical activity on insulin sensitivity. A high frequency of weekly physical activity can be maintained by using a combination of workout intensities, such that lower intensities are utilized on "recovery days" following higher-intensity workout days. If individuals with pre-diabetes are able to perform both aerobic and resistance physical activity, they should be encouraged to adopt both types of exercise to receive the overlapping and complementary effects on insulin sensitivity and glycemic control [65].

4. Sleep and influence of sleep patterns on insulin regulation

Sleep is a periodic, consciously controlled state of reduced awareness, relaxed muscles, and changed reaction to stimuli and it is believed that sleep is harmless [66]. Adequate sleep is necessary for vital functions and overall health while lack of sleep has an impact on immune system performance, mood, autonomic nervous system activity, and attentiveness [67].

Changes in insulin sensitivity and production, which control glucose homeostasis, lead to T2DM. Sleep and normal glucose homeostasis are related. Insulin and plasma glucose production are increased during early nocturnal sleep, but they revert to pre-sleep levels during late sleep. Insulin and glucose secretion are dramatically changed by sleep loss. In that case, even with bed rest, they stay steady for the first part of the night before dropping off significantly. Six in a 24-hour cycle involving continuous enteral feeding, Simon et al. [68] investigated whether the ultradian and circadian glucose and insulin secretion rates of eight night shift workers responded to a permanent nocturnal schedule. Eight-day active participants with nocturnal and acute 8-hour shifting sleep were compared to these subjects. Insulin and glucose secretion rates in patients who were awake during the daytime shifted from high levels throughout the night to low levels during the poor night and daytime sleep that followed the acute sleep transition. The glucose rise only shifted 6 hours with the sleep shift in night shift workers, and the sleep-related amplification of the oscillations did not happen simultaneously. Instead, the peak levels of the glucose and insulin secretion rates shifted 8 hours with the sleep shift.

In another significant 1999 work, Spiegel et al. investigated the effects of six nights of 4-hour sleep restriction on glucose metabolism as assessed by intravenous glucose tolerance testing (IVGTT) [69]. When compared to a fully rested 12-hour TIB condition, a 4-hour sleep restriction resulted in a 24% decrease in insulin sensitivity and a 30% decrease in acute insulin response to glucose, suggesting an inadequate β-cell response to developing insulin resistance [69, 70]. This decline in insulin sensitivity was comparable to both gestational diabetes and aging. Heart sympatho-vagal activity was unbalanced, favoring greater sympathetic tone, in addition to alterations in glucose metabolism. The 24-hour cortisol profile revealed higher afternoon and evening levels.

4.1 Sleep restriction and insulin resistance: possible mechanism

Numerous physiological processes, including as muscle insulin resistance, adipocyte function, and the release of insulin and glucagon, are impacted by sympathetic nervous system activity [71]. Moreover, one possible contributing factor is activation of the hypothalamic-pituitary-adrenal (HPA) axis. Studies on sleep loss have shown a potential link between increases in cortisol levels in the afternoon and evening and insulin resistance. Insulin resistance in the morning can be exacerbated by GH secretion at night following sleep restriction [72, 73]. Increased inflammatory markers have also been linked to sleep deprivation [74]. Among them are hsCRP, TNF-α, IL-1β, IL-6, IL-17, and elevated leukocytes and monocytes [71]. Insulin resistance is linked to the markers [75]. Adipocyte dysfunction is now associated with sleep deprivation and metabolic problems. "Adipocyte insulin resistance" may result from sympathetic nervous system activity and HPA axis activation. Four nights without sleep decreased adipocyte insulin signaling by 30%, according to research by [76]. Insulin sensitivity throughout the body decreased, according to IVGTT. Insulin resistance may increase as a result of lipolysis and NEFA release brought on by reduced insulin signaling in adipocytes [71]. Insulin sensitivity dropped and fasting and 24-hour NEFA increased in many sleep restriction experiments [73]. These changes may possibly be involved because the rise in nighttime NEFA was found to be strongly correlated with longer GH and higher levels of adrenaline in the early morning [73]. A lack of sleep has an impact on hormones that control hunger, food intake, and energy expenditure. These factors may have an indirect effect on the metabolism of glucose and the risk of developing diabetes by promoting weight gain and insulin resistance.

4.2 Sleep hygiene to enhance the quality and duration of sleep

Good sleep enhances both physical and mental well-being and increases productivity. Everyone, from young children to elderly people, may benefit from good sleep hygiene. Excellent habits are critical to health, according to research [77]. Good habits become almost instinctual via the development of enduring and advantageous routines that provide continuous reinforcement. Even if harmful habits are bad for you, they may nonetheless become ingrained.

A regular sleep schedule in sync with the circadian rhythm is necessary to optimize insulin management. Sleep rhythm is supported by a regular wake-up time on the weekends and throughout the week. Sleep should be prioritized, even when faced with tempting activities like work, study, or socializing. It is advisable to calculate a target bedtime based on the fixed wake-up time and make it a priority to be ready for bed around that time each night. If there is a need to shift sleep times, gradual adjustments should be made in small steps, up to an hour or two, to avoid disrupting the schedule. Napping can be useful for energy boosters, but keeping them short and limited to the early afternoon helps prevent interference with nighttime sleep. Creating an optimal sleep environment involves factors like darkness and temperature, which support hormonal regulation and enhance sleep quality [78, 79].

Having a comfortable mattress and pillow, using excellent bedding, setting a cool yet comfortable temperature, blocking out light, drowning out noise, and trying calming scents contribute to a peaceful sleep environment. Reducing screen time before bed helps insulin regulation and melatonin production in accordance with circadian rhythms. The body relaxes when it engages in circadian sleep habits like reading or resting.

To reduce disruptions to sleep, avoiding large meals and caffeine close to bedtime should align with circadian metabolic processes. Reducing stress at night enhances insulin sensitivity, demonstrating the connection between stress and metabolic well-being. Exercise earlier in the day is beneficial since it may improve insulin regulation late in the day [78, 79]. Insulin sensitivity, sleep-wake cycles, and circadian rhythms are all regulated by sunlight, particularly in the morning. These strategies focus on aligning lifestyle decisions with circadian principles to improve metabolic health and insulin regulation.

5. Stress and role of stress in insulin resistance

Stress is defined as a state of altered body homeostasis brought on by somatic stressors such as, nutritional deprivation, viral infections, chemical toxins, ischemia, heat shock, inflammation and lipid accumulation as well as psychological causes such as depression, worry, and fear. Any of these may result in physiological alterations that support the organism's survival and equilibrium [80]. Stress affects the CNS and peripheral neuroendocrine systems, which are intricate systems. The primary hormonal effectors of the stress system are glucocorticoids and catecholaminas, which are ultimate mediators of the hypothalamic-pituitary-adrenal-axis and sympathetic nervous system. Hormones associated with chronic stress can alter glucose homeostasis, whereas acute stress may not. Acute stress, in particular, raises insulin secretion and glucose concentration, which promotes glucose clearance and preserves normoglycemia. Allostatic processes are triggered by ongoing stresses. The phrase "glucose allostasis" was first used by Ref. [81] to describe the mechanism wherein glucose levels stay raised after prolonged stress, thereby warning the β-cell of insulin resistance. This causes T2DM and elevated glycemia even in the presence of normal beta-cell function.

Glucocorticoids are so named due to their impact on glucose metabolism [82]. The body uses all of its energy reserves to maintain homeostasis when glucocorticoids stimulate the liver's gluconeogenesis and glycogen storage. Furthermore, glucocorticoids decrease the absorption and use of glucose in white adipose tissue and skeletal muscle, leading to hyperglycemia—the most prevalent and quickly aggravating adverse impact of drug usage and hyperstimulation [82–84]. Hypercortisolemia brought on by prolonged stress may cause insulin resistance, visceral obesity, and a reduction in lean body mass. The liver produces more glucose as a direct consequence of glucocorticoids' stimulation of glucose-6-phosphatase and phosphoenolpyruvate carboxykinase. The metabolism of insulin is indirectly hampered by glucocorticoids [85]. Glucocorticoids promote the liver's synthesis of glucose via acting on glucagon and adrenaline [82]. Glucocorticoids counteract the effects of insulin signaling by decreasing the absorption of glucose in peripheral tissue and skeletal muscle.

Insulin-dependent peripheral glucose absorption is regulated by a transporter called GLUT 4 [86]. Insulin increases the expression of this transporter, which is mostly found in skeletal muscle. In these tissues, GLUT 4 is expressed more when glucocorticoids are present, but they also stop it from moving to the cell surface in response to insulin and other stimuli (including hypoxia) [85]. As a consequence, when glucose is consumed, less of it is absorbed. Glucocorticoids cause white adipose tissue to undergo lypolisis, which produces glycerol needed for the gluconeogenic process. As a consequence, non-esterified fatty acids build up in muscle cells, interfering with insulin signaling and preventing the absorption and use of glucose. Insulin synthesis and β-cell secretion are impeded by the pancreatic presence of costicosteroids [86].

A prolonged period of stress may heighten the sympathetic nervous system's activity, which can lower glucose tolerance and raise the risk of an acute cardiovascular event [87]. The body responds to catecholamine infusion by increasing gluconeogenesis, glycolysis, and glycogenolysis [88]. It could prevent insulin from facilitating glycogenesis, which would cause hyperglycemia and hyperlactatemia. Insulin resistance can be brought on by epinephrine, norepinephrine, and β adrenergic receptor (AR) activation [89]. In adipocytes, the β3 AR triggers hormone-sensitive lipase, which results in the build-up of free fatty acids, heightened MAPK activation, and the production of ceramides [90]. By inhibiting the activity of protein kinase B (PKB), ceramide exacerbates insulin resistance [91]. Increased insulin resistance in tissues is a result of all the processes mentioned above, and in these patients, type II diabetes can develop.

5.1 Mindfulness practice and meditation as tools for stress reduction

Purposeful, nonjudgmental focus on the present is what is meant by mindfulness. It entails having an inquiring, receptive, and welcoming attitude toward one's present feelings, ideas, physical experiences, and environment [92]. Mindfulness is developed by meditation, which focuses on breathing, bodily sensations, a thought, or a phrase. Numerous studies have been conducted on the advantages of mindfulness for reducing stress, mental health, well-being, and cognitive performance [93]. In MBSR and MBCT, mindfulness exercises are often used. The goal of these treatments is to support patients in controlling their feelings, thoughts, and mental health [94]. Additionally, studies have shown that mindfulness therapies help diabetics with their chronic pain, insulin resistance, irritable bowel syndrome symptoms, and glycemic management [95]. Enhancing attention, mood, and self-awareness with mindfulness may help control CVD risk variables such physical activity, medication adherence, smoking, and nutrition [96].

Yoga, an ancient Indian practice, has demonstrated promising glycemic control in T2DM patients [97, 98]. Yoga practice consists of two components: physical activity (postures/asana) and relaxation (meditation, shavasana). Yoga, with its emphasis on breath control, posture holding, and meditation, helps practitioners focus on body sensations and present-moment experiences. This state of nonjudgment and attention to one's present experiences contributes to yoga's mindfulness-based nature [99]. This may help with diabetes management because mindfulness training has been shown to improve one's ability to recognize and respond to emotional stress, resulting in effective coping responses [100].

It is yet unclear how mindfulness affects physical health at its fundamental level. Three pathways make up its mechanism of action, according to Creswell et al. [92]: biological, health behavior, and psychological. The biological mechanism is one of the most important in figuring out how mindfulness affects glucose metabolism among them. Controlling the prefrontal cortex's stress regulation areas (also known as the regulatory route) and the brain's stress alarm system (also known as the reactivity pathway) is the main physiologic impact of mindfulness. Prior studies have demonstrated that mindfulness therapies can alter the autonomic nervous system (ANS) and the hypothalamic-pituitary-adrenal (HPA) axis in response to external stress, as well as lower interleukin (IL)-6 levels in stressed individuals [95].

6. Conclusion

This book chapter explores the complex relationships between lifestyle factors and insulin sensitivity. The elements of stress management, exercise, sleep, and diet are given special consideration. Many well accepted notions about diet are questioned, and the effects of high sugar and specific fats on insulin resistance are shown. It has been shown that eating entire foods, especially plant-based diets, may improve insulin sensitivity via a variety of biochemical pathways. It focuses on the molecular mechanisms by which exercise increases insulin sensitivity. This study examines the role that exercise—which encompasses both strength and aerobic training—plays. Even though it is sometimes disregarded, sleep is well recognized as a factor that affects insulin regulation. This chapter examines the potential effects of stress—both psychological and physical—on insulin resistance, focusing in particular on stress hormones. The last section of the chapter looks at mindfulness and meditation as potential methods for controlling insulin resistance and lowering stress. This makes it hard to overstate the importance of treating and preventing metabolic illnesses with a comprehensive strategy that takes into account all of these interconnected lifestyle factors.

Author details

Olorunfemi Oyewole Babalola[1*], Paul Olamide Ottu[1], Ebenezer Akinnusi[1], Precious Olayinka Aturamu[1] and Opeyemi Iwaloye[2]

1 Department of Chemical Sciences, Biochemistry Unit, Olusegun Agagu University of Science and Technology Okitipupa, Okitipupa, Nigeria

2 Department of Biochemistry, Federal University of Technology Akure, Akure, Nigeria

*Address all correspondence to: babalolaolorunfemi20@gmail.com

IntechOpen

References

[1] Lema-Pérez L. Main organs involved in glucose metabolism. In: Sugar Intake-Risks and Benefits and the Global Diabetes Epidemic. London, UK: IntechOpen; 2021

[2] DeFronzo RA. From the triumvirate to the ominous octet: A new paradigm for the treatment of type 2 diabetes mellitus. Diabetes. 2009;**58**(4):773-795

[3] Taylor R. Insulin resistance and type 2 diabetes. Diabetes. 2012;**61**(4):778

[4] Eckel RH, Kahn SE, Ferrannini E, Goldfine AB, Nathan DM, Schwartz MW, et al. Obesity and type 2 diabetes: What can be unified and what needs to be individualized? The Journal of Clinical Endocrinology & Metabolism. 2011;**96**(6):1654-1663

[5] Reaven GM. Insulin resistance: The link between obesity and cardiovascular disease. Endocrinology and Metabolism Clinics of North America. 2008;**37**(3):581-601

[6] Rodriguez-Gutierrez R, Gonzalez-Gonzalez JG, Zuñiga-Hernandez JA, McCoy RG. Benefits and harms of intensive glycemic control in patients with type 2 diabetes. BMJ. 2019. pp. 158-187

[7] Unwin D, Livesey G, Haslam D. It is the glycaemic response to, not the carbohydrate content of food that matters in diabetes and obesity: The glycaemic index revisited. Journal of Insulin Resistance. 2016;**1**(1):1-9

[8] Yang W, Jiang W, Guo S. Regulation of macronutrients in insulin resistance and glucose homeostasis during type 2 diabetes mellitus. Nutrients. 2023;**15**(21):4671

[9] Stanhope KL. Sugar consumption, metabolic disease and obesity: The state of the controversy. Critical Reviews in Clinical Laboratory Sciences. 2016;**53**(1):52-67

[10] Tappy L, Lê KA. Metabolic effects of fructose and the worldwide increase in obesity. Physiological Reviews. 2010;**90**(1):23-46

[11] Jensen T, Abdelmalek MF, Sullivan S, Nadeau KJ, Green M, Roncal C, et al. Fructose and sugar: A major mediator of non-alcoholic fatty liver disease. Journal of Hepatology. 2018;**68**(5):1063-1075

[12] Riccardi G, Rivellese AA. Dietary treatment of the metabolic syndrome—The optimal diet. British Journal of Nutrition. 2000;**83**(S1):S143-S148

[13] Montgomery MK, Osborne B, Brown SH, Small L, Mitchell TW, Cooney GJ, et al. Contrasting metabolic effects of medium-versus long-chain fatty acids in skeletal muscle. Journal of Lipid Research. 2013;**54**(12):3322-3333

[14] Canfora EE, Jocken JW, Blaak EE. Short-chain fatty acids in control of body weight and insulin sensitivity. Nature Reviews Endocrinology. 2015;**11**(10):577-591

[15] Parillo M, Riccardi G. Diet composition and the risk of type 2 diabetes: Epidemiological and clinical evidence. British Journal of Nutrition. 2004;**92**(1):7-19

[16] Fock KM, Khoo J. Diet and exercise in management of obesity and overweight. Journal of Gastroenterology and Hepatology. 2013;**28**:59-63

[17] McClenaghan NH. Determining the relationship between dietary carbohydrate intake and insulin resistance. Nutrition Research Reviews. 2005;**18**(2):222-240

[18] Lundsgaard AM, Holm JB, Sjøberg KA, Bojsen-Møller KN, Myrmel LS, Fjære E, et al. Mechanisms preserving insulin action during high dietary fat intake. Cell Metabolism. 2019;**29**(1):50-63

[19] Messina M, Sievenpiper JL, Williamson P, Kiel J, Erdman JW Jr. Perspective: Soy-based meat and dairy alternatives, despite classification as ultra-processed foods, deliver high-quality nutrition on par with unprocessed or minimally processed animal-based counterparts. Advances in Nutrition. 2022;**13**(3):726-738

[20] De la Iglesia R, Loria-Kohen V, Zulet MA, Martinez JA, Reglero G, Ramirez de Molina A. Dietary strategies implicated in the prevention and treatment of metabolic syndrome. International Journal of Molecular Sciences. 2016;**17**(11):1877

[21] Malik VS, Hu FB. Sugar-sweetened beverages and cardiometabolic health: An update of the evidence. Nutrients. 2019;**11**(8):1840

[22] Arabzadegan N, Daneshzad E, Fatahi S, Moosavian SP, Surkan PJ, Azadbakht L. Effects of dietary whole grain, fruit, and vegetables on weight and inflammatory biomarkers in overweight and obese women. Eating and Weight Disorders-Studies on Anorexia, Bulimia and Obesity. 2020;**25**:1243-1251

[23] Wallace TC, Bailey RL, Blumberg JB, Burton-Freeman B, Chen CO, Crowe-White KM, et al. Fruits, vegetables, and health: A comprehensive narrative, umbrella review of the science and recommendations for enhanced public policy to improve intake. Critical Reviews in Food Science and Nutrition. 2020;**60**(13):2174-2211

[24] Wallace IR, McEvoy CT, Hunter SJ, Hamill LL, Ennis CN, Bell PM, et al. Dose-response effect of fruit and vegetables on insulin resistance in people at high risk of cardiovascular disease: A randomized controlled trial. Diabetes Care. 2013;**36**(12):3888-3896

[25] Wang W, Liu Y, Li Y, Luo B, Lin Z, Chen K, et al. Dietary patterns and cardiometabolic health: Clinical evidence and mechanism. MedComm. 2023;**4**(1):e212

[26] Fujii H, Iwase M, Ohkuma T, Ogata-Kaizu S, Ide H, Kikuchi Y, et al. Impact of dietary fiber intake on glycemic control, cardiovascular risk factors and chronic kidney disease in Japanese patients with type 2 diabetes mellitus: The Fukuoka diabetes registry. Nutrition Journal. 2023;**12**:159. DOI: 10.1186/1475-2891-12-159

[27] Zhang P. Influence of foods and nutrition on the gut microbiome and implications for intestinal health. International Journal of Molecular Sciences. 2022;**23**(17):9588

[28] García-García FJ, Monistrol-Mula A, Cardellach F, Garrabou G. Nutrition, bioenergetics, and metabolic syndrome. Nutrients. 2020;**12**(9):2785

[29] Číž M, Dvořáková A, Skočková V, Kubala L. The role of dietary phenolic compounds in epigenetic modulation involved in inflammatory processes. Antioxidants. 2020;**9**(8):691

[30] Cowan SF, Leeming ER, Sinclair A, Dordevic AL, Truby H, Gibson SJ. Effect of whole foods and dietary patterns on markers of subclinical inflammation

in weight-stable overweight and obese adults: A systematic review. Nutrition Reviews. 2020;**78**(1):19-38

[31] Hawley JA. Exercise as a therapeutic intervention for the prevention and treatment of insulin resistance. Diabetes/metabolism Research and Reviews. 2004;**20**(5):383-393

[32] Balducci S, Sacchetti M, Haxhi J, Orlando G, D'Errico V, Fallucca S, et al. Physical exercise as therapy for type 2 diabetes mellitus. Diabetes/metabolism Research and Reviews. 2014;**30**(S1):13-23

[33] Thaane T, Motala AA, McKune AJ. Effects of short-term exercise in overweight/obese adults with insulin resistance or type 2 diabetes: A systematic review of randomized controlled trials. Journal of Diabetes & Metabolism. 2018;**9**(12):816

[34] Pearson MJ, Mungovan SF, Smart NA. Effect of aerobic and resistance training on inflammatory markers in heart failure patients: Systematic review and meta-analysis. Heart Failure Reviews. 2018;**23**:209-223

[35] Makki K, Froguel P, Wolowczuk I. Adipose tissue in obesity-related inflammation and insulin resistance: Cells, cytokines, and chemokines. ISRN Inflammation; 2013. pp. 1-12

[36] Yavari A, Najafipoor F, Aliasgarzadeh A, Niafar M, Mobasseri M. Effect of aerobic exercise, resistance training or combined training on glycaemic control and cardio-vascular risk factors in patients with type 2 diabetes. Biology of Sport. 2012;**29**(2):135-143

[37] Kohut ML, McCann DA, Russell DW, Konopka DN, Cunnick JE, Franke WD, et al. Aerobic exercise, but not flexibility/resistance exercise, reduces serum IL-18, CRP, and IL-6 independent of β-blockers, BMI, and psychosocial factors in older adults. Brain, Behavior, and Immunity. 2006;**20**(3):201-209

[38] Abd El-Kader SM. Aerobic versus resistance exercise training in modulation of insulin resistance, adipocytokines and inflammatory cytokine levels in obese type 2 diabetic patients. Journal of Advanced Research. 2011;**2**(2):179-183

[39] Dekker MJ, Lee S, Hudson R, Kilpatrick K, Graham TE, Ross R, et al. An exercise intervention without weight loss decreases circulating interleukin-6 in lean and obese men with and without type 2 diabetes mellitus. Metabolism. 2007;**56**(3):332-338

[40] Henriksen EJ. Invited review: Effects of acute exercise and exercise training on insulin resistance. Journal of Applied Physiology. 2002;**93**(2):788-796

[41] Burr JF, Rowan CP, Jamnik VK, Riddell MC. The role of physical activity in type 2 diabetes prevention: Physiological and practical perspectives. The Physician and Sportsmedicine. 2010;**38**(1):72-82

[42] Borghouts LB, Keizer HA. Exercise and insulin sensitivity: A review. International Journal of Sports Medicine. 2000;**21**(01):1-2

[43] Imierska M, Kurianiuk A, Błachnio-Zabielska A. The influence of physical activity on the bioactive lipids metabolism in obesity-induced muscle insulin resistance. Biomolecules. 2020;**10**(12):1665

[44] Willis LH, Slentz CA, Bateman LA, Shields AT, Piner LW, Bales CW, et al. Effects of aerobic and/or resistance training on body mass and fat mass

in overweight or obese adults. Journal of Applied Physiology. 2012;**113**(12):1831-1837

[45] Sung KD, Pekas EJ, Scott SD, Son WM, Park SY. The effects of a 12-week jump rope exercise program on abdominal adiposity, vasoactive substances, inflammation, and vascular function in adolescent girls with prehypertension. European Journal of Applied Physiology. 2019;**119**:577-585

[46] Tilg H, Moschen AR. Adipocytokines: Mediators linking adipose tissue, inflammation and immunity. Nature Reviews Immunology. 2006;**6**(10):772-783

[47] Lumeng CN, Saltiel AR. Inflammatory links between obesity and metabolic disease. The Journal of Clinical Investigation. 2011;**121**(6):2111-2117

[48] Olefsky JM, Glass CK. Macrophages, inflammation, and insulin resistance. Annual Review of Physiology. 2010;**72**:219-246

[49] Chang C, Liu W, Zhao X, Li S, Yu C. Effect of supervised exercise intervention on metabolic risk factors and physical fitness in Chinese obese children in early puberty. Obesity Reviews. 2008;**9**:135-141

[50] Shaibi GQ, Cruz ML, Ball GD, Weigensberg MJ, Salem GJ, Crespo NC, et al. Effects of resistance training on insulin sensitivity in overweight Latino adolescent males. Medicine and Science in Sports and Exercise. 2006;**38**(7):1208

[51] Davis JN, Gyllenhammer LE, Vanni AA, Meija M, Tung A, Schroeder ET, et al. Startup circuit training program reduces metabolic risk in Latino adolescents. Medicine and Science in Sports and Exercise. 2011;**43**(11):2195

[52] Lee S, Libman I, Hughan K, Kuk JL, Jeong JH, Zhang D, et al. Effects of exercise modality on insulin resistance and ectopic fat in adolescents with overweight and obesity: A randomized clinical trial. The Journal of Pediatrics. 2019;**206**:91-98

[53] Wong PC, Chia MY, Tsou IY, Wansaicheong GK, Tan B, Wang JC, et al. Effects of a 12-week exercise training programme on aerobic fitness, body composition, blood lipids and C-reactive protein in adolescents with obesity. Annals Academy of Medicine Singapore. 1 Apr 2008;**37**(4):286

[54] Bell LM, Watts K, Siafarikas A, Thompson A, Ratnam N, Bulsara M, et al. Exercise alone reduces insulin resistance in obese children independently of changes in body composition. The Journal of Clinical Endocrinology & Metabolism. 2007;**92**(11):4230-4235

[55] Ren JM, Semenkovich CF, Gulve EA, Gao J, Holloszy JO. Exercise induces rapid increases in GLUT4 expression, glucose transport capacity, and insulin-stimulated glycogen storage in muscle. Journal of Biological Chemistry. 1994;**269**(20):14396-14401

[56] Bradley H, Shaw CS, Bendtsen C, Worthington PL, Wilson OJ, Strauss JA, et al. Visualization and quantitation of GLUT 4 translocation in human skeletal muscle following glucose ingestion and exercise. Physiological Reports. 2015;**3**(5):e12375

[57] Russell AP. PGC-1α and exercise: Important partners in combating insulin resistance. Current Diabetes Reviews. 2005;**1**(2):175-181

[58] Sangwung P, Petersen KF, Shulman GI, Knowles JW. Mitochondrial dysfunction, insulin resistance, and

potential genetic implications: Potential role of alterations in mitochondrial function in the pathogenesis of insulin resistance and type 2 diabetes. Endocrinology. 2020;**161**(4):bqaa017

[59] Gutiérrez-Rodelo C, Roura-Guiberna A, Olivares-Reyes JA. Molecular mechanisms of insulin resistance: An update. Gaceta Médica de México. 2017;**153**(2):214-218

[60] Basciano H, Federico L, Adeli K. Fructose, insulin resistance, and metabolic dyslipidemia. Nutrition & Metabolism. 2005;**2**(1):1-4

[61] Etnier JL, Nowell PM, Landers DM, Sibley BA. A meta-regression to examine the relationship between aerobic fitness and cognitive performance. Brain Research Reviews. 2006;**52**(1):119-130

[62] Nikolaidis MG, Jamurtas AZ, Paschalis V, Fatouros IG, Koutedakis Y, Kouretas D. The effect of muscle-damaging exercise on blood and skeletal muscle oxidative stress: Magnitude and time-course considerations. Sports Medicine. 2008;**38**:579-606

[63] Barzilay J. The pre-diabetic, insulin-resistant state. The Epidemiology of Aging. 2012:433-452

[64] Vissers D, Hens W, Taeymans J, Baeyens JP, Poortmans J, Van Gaal L. The effect of exercise on visceral adipose tissue in overweight adults: A systematic review and meta-analysis. PLoS One. 2013;**8**(2):e56415

[65] Runge-Morris M, Kocarek TA, Falany CN. Regulation of the cytosolic sulfotransferases by nuclear receptors. Drug Metabolism Reviews. 2013;**45**(1): 15-33

[66] Saleh SA. Sleep and dreaming. In: The Psychology of Consciousness: Theory and Practice. Cham: Springer International Publishing; 2022. pp. 39-56

[67] Medic G, Wille M, Hemels ME. Short-and long-term health consequences of sleep disruption. Nature and Science of Sleep. 2017;**9**:151-161

[68] Simon C, Weibel L, Brandenberger G. Twenty-four-hour rhythms of plasma glucose and insulin secretion rate in regular night workers. American Journal of Physiology-Endocrinology and Metabolism. 2000;**278**(3):E413-E420

[69] Spiegel K, Leproult R, Van Cauter E. Impact of sleep debt on metabolic and endocrine function. The Lancet. 1999;**354**(9188):1435-1439

[70] Leproult R, Van Cauter E. Role of sleep and sleep loss in hormonal release and metabolism. Pediatric Neuroendocrinology. 2010;**17**:11-21

[71] Reutrakul S, Van Cauter E. Sleep influences on obesity, insulin resistance, and risk of type 2 diabetes. Metabolism. 2018;**84**:56-66

[72] Buxton OM, Pavlova M, Reid EW, Wang W, Simonson DC, Adler GK. Sleep restriction for 1 week reduces insulin sensitivity in healthy men. Diabetes. 2010;**59**(9):2126-2133

[73] Broussard JL, Chapotot F, Abraham V, Day A, Delebecque F, Whitmore HR, et al. Sleep restriction increases free fatty acids in healthy men. Diabetologia. 2015;**58**:791-798

[74] Faraut B, Boudjeltia KZ, Vanhamme L, Kerkhofs M. Immune, inflammatory and cardiovascular consequences of sleep restriction and recovery. Sleep Medicine Reviews. 2012;**16**(2):137-149

[75] Wieser V, Moschen AR, Tilg H. Inflammation, cytokines and insulin resistance: A clinical perspective. Archivum Immunologiae et Therapiae Experimentalis. 2013;**61**:119-125

[76] Broussard JL, Ehrmann DA, Van Cauter E, Tasali E, Brady MJ. Impaired insulin signaling in human adipocytes after experimental sleep restriction: A randomized, crossover study. Annals of Internal Medicine. 2012;**157**(8):549-557

[77] Harmsen JF, Wefers J, Doligkeit D, Schlangen L, Dautzenberg B, Rense P, et al. The influence of bright and dim light on substrate metabolism, energy expenditure and thermoregulation in insulin-resistant individuals depends on time of day. Diabetologia. 2022;**65**(4):721-732

[78] Ruddick-Collins LC, Morgan PJ, Johnstone AM. Mealtime: A circadian disruptor and determinant of energy balance? Journal of Neuroendocrinology. 2020;**32**(7):e12886

[79] Zhang K, Ma Y, Luo Y, Song Y, Xiong G, Ma Y, et al. Metabolic diseases and healthy aging: Identifying environmental and behavioral risk factors and promoting public health. Frontiers in Public Health. 13 Oct 2023;**11**:1253506

[80] Tsiotra PC, Tsigos C. Stress, the endoplasmic reticulum, and insulin resistance. Annals of the New York Academy of Sciences. 2006;**1083**(1):63-76

[81] Stumvoll M, Tataranni PA, Stefan N, Vozarova B, Bogardus C. Glucose allostasis. Diabetes. 2003;**52**(4):903-909

[82] Kuo T, McQueen A, Chen TC, Wang JC. Regulation of Glucose Homeostasis by Glucocorticoids. Glucocorticoid Signaling. 2015. pp. 99-126

[83] Perez A, Jansen-Chaparro S, Saigi I, Bernal-Lopez MR, Miñambres I, Gomez-Huelgas R. Glucocorticoid-induced hyperglycemia. Journal of Diabetes. 2014;**6**(1):9-20

[84] Hwang JL, Weiss RE. Steroid-induced diabetes: A clinical and molecular approach to understanding and treatment. Diabetes/metabolism Research and Reviews. 2014;**30**(2):96-102

[85] Ingrosso DM, Primavera M, Samvelyan S, Tagi VM, Chiarelli F. Stress and diabetes mellitus: Pathogenetic mechanisms and clinical outcome. Hormone Research in Paediatrics. 2023;**96**(1):34-43

[86] Kuo T, Harris CA, Wang JC. Metabolic functions of glucocorticoid receptor in skeletal muscle. Molecular and Cellular Endocrinology. 2013;**380**(1-2):79-88

[87] Rozanski A, Blumenthal JA, Kaplan J. Impact of psychological factors on the pathogenesis of cardiovascular disease and implications for therapy. Circulation. 1999;**99**(16):2192-2217

[88] Barth E, Albuszies G, Baumgart K, Matejovic M, Wachter U, Vogt J, et al. Glucose metabolism and catecholamines. Critical Care Medicine. 2007;**35**(9):S508-S518

[89] Onyango AN. Cellular stresses and stress responses in the pathogenesis of insulin resistance. Oxidative Medicine and Cellular Longevity. 2018;**2018**:1-27

[90] Mottillo EP, Shen XJ, Granneman JG. β3-adrenergic receptor induction of adipocyte inflammation requires lipolytic activation of stress kinases p38 and JNK. Biochimica et Biophysica Acta

(BBA)-Molecular and Cell Biology of Lipids. 2010;**1801**(9):1048-1055

[91] Reali F, Morine MJ, Kahramanoğulları O, Raichur S, Schneider HC, Crowther D, et al. Mechanistic interplay between ceramide and insulin resistance. Scientific Reports. 2017;**7**(1):41231

[92] Creswell JD, Lindsay EK, Villalba DK, Chin B. Mindfulness training and physical health: Mechanisms and outcomes. Psychosomatic Medicine. 2019;**81**(3):224

[93] Zhang D, Lee EK, Mak EC, Ho CY, Wong SY. Mindfulness-based interventions: An overall review. British Medical Bulletin. 2021;**138**(1):41-57

[94] Alsubaie M, Abbott R, Dunn B, Dickens C, Keil TF, Henley W, et al. Mechanisms of action in mindfulness-based cognitive therapy (MBCT) and mindfulness-based stress reduction (MBSR) in people with physical and/or psychological conditions: A systematic review. Clinical Psychology Review. 2017;**55**:74-91

[95] Loucks EB, Schuman-Olivier Z, Britton WB, Fresco DM, Desbordes G, Brewer JA, et al. Mindfulness and cardiovascular disease risk: State of the evidence, plausible mechanisms, and theoretical framework. Current Cardiology Reports. 2015;**17**:1-1

[96] Tang YY, Hölzel BK, Posner MI. The neuroscience of mindfulness meditation. Nature Reviews Neuroscience. 2015;**16**(4):213-225

[97] Kumar V, Jagannathan A, Philip M, Thulasi A, Angadi P, Raghuram N. Role of yoga for patients with type II diabetes mellitus: A systematic review and meta-analysis. Complementary Therapies in Medicine. 2016;**25**:104-112

[98] Cui J, Yan JH, Yan LM, Pan L, Le JJ, Guo YZ. Effects of yoga in adults with type 2 diabetes mellitus: A meta-analysis. Journal of Diabetes Investigation. 2017;**8**(2):201-209

[99] Kabat-Zinn J. Mindfulness-based interventions in context: past, present, and future. Clinical Psychology: Science and Practice. 2003;**10**(2):144-156

[100] Vago DR, Silbersweig DA. Self-awareness, self-regulation, and self-transcendence (S-ART): A framework for understanding the neurobiological mechanisms of mindfulness. Frontiers in Human Neuroscience. 2012;**6**:296

Chapter 9

Exploring the Function of Inflammatory Routes in Insulin Resistance: Interpreting the Inflammatory Veil of Medusa

Anchala Kumari

Abstract

A common component of metabolic diseases including metabolic syndrome and type 2 diabetes, insulin resistance is now known to be closely linked to persistent low-grade inflammation. This chapter explores the intricate connection between insulin resistance and inflammatory pathways, clarifying the molecular processes that underlie inflammation-induced insulin resistance. We examine the part that important inflammatory mediators play in upsetting insulin signalling pathways and encouraging insulin resistance, including cytokines, chemokines, and adipokines. We also go over how inflammatory signalling cascades, like the JNK and NF-κB pathways, affect insulin sensitivity and cellular metabolism. Understanding the interaction between insulin resistance and inflammation can help to better understand the pathogenesis of metabolic diseases and identify possible treatment targets. In people who are at risk of developing issues associated with insulin resistance, strategies targeted at reducing inflammatory responses may be able to reduce insulin resistance and enhance metabolic health.

Keywords: insulin resistance, metabolic syndrome, type 2 diabetes, Medusa, inflammation

1. Introduction

Insulin resistance (IR) is a major contributor to the pathophysiology of metabolic diseases, such as metabolic syndrome and type 2 diabetes mellitus (T2DM), and it has a substantial impact on global health. According to newly available data, insulin resistance develops and progresses as a result of a complex interplay between inflammatory and metabolic pathways and persistent low-grade inflammation. Insulin resistance has many facets, and the idea that it is the "Medusa of the 21st Century" effectively conveys this. One of its veils is inflammation, which obscures its underlying mechanisms.

Several studies have demonstrated the connection between inflammation and insulin resistance, linking inflammatory mediators to insulin signalling pathway disruption

IntechOpen

and glucose homeostasis impairment [1, 2]. These mediators include cytokines, chemokines, and adipokines. Among them, interleukin-6 (IL-6), adiponectin, and tumour necrosis factor-alpha (TNF-α) have become important participants in the inflammatory cascade, influencing insulin sensitivity both locally and systemically [3, 4].

Furthermore, complex signalling pathways, such as c-Jun N-terminal kinase (JNK) and nuclear factor kappa B (NF-κB), facilitate the interaction between insulin resistance and inflammation, causing metabolic processes to become dysregulated and accelerating the development of metabolic diseases [5, 6]. Insulin receptor substrate (IRS) proteins get phosphorylated when these pro-inflammatory pathways are activated, upsetting insulin signalling cascades and ultimately resulting in insulin resistance [7].

To reduce inflammation and restore metabolic balance, specific therapeutic approaches that comprehend the molecular pathways behind inflammation-induced insulin resistance are necessary. We can create individualised strategies for treating insulin resistance and its related problems by dissecting the intricacies of this complicated interaction.

We explore the role of inflammatory pathways in insulin resistance in this chapter, looking at the molecular mechanisms through which inflammation fuels insulin resistance and the consequences for metabolic health. We seek to clarify the inflammatory veil that covers Medusa and provide insight into prospective targets and tactics for treating insulin resistance-related illnesses by conducting a thorough analysis of recent literature and emerging research discoveries.

2. Literature review

The pathophysiology of insulin resistance and related metabolic problems is largely dependent on persistent low-grade inflammation, as demonstrated by a large number of studies. Clarifying the processes behind inflammation-induced insulin resistance and discovering possible treatment targets require an understanding of the complex interactions between inflammatory mediators and signalling pathways.

TNF-α has been identified as a crucial mediator between inflammation and insulin resistance. Through the activation of serine kinases including c-Jun N-terminal kinase (JNK) and IκB kinase (IKK), which phosphorylate insulin receptor substrate (IRS) proteins and interfere with downstream insulin signalling, TNF-α has been shown in experimental experiments to block insulin signalling pathways [1, 2]. Clinical research has demonstrated increased TNF-α levels in patients with type 2 diabetes mellitus (T2DM) and obesity, further linking TNF-α to the aetiology of insulin resistance [2, 8].

Another pro-inflammatory cytokine linked to the emergence of insulin resistance is interleukin-6 (IL-6). Research has indicated that persistent increase in IL-6 levels impedes insulin signalling and glucose absorption in skeletal muscle, which in turn leads to insulin resistance [9, 10]. Acute-phase proteins like C-reactive protein (CRP), which worsen insulin resistance and prolong the inflammatory response, are also secreted in greater amounts when IL-6 is present [11].

Adiponectin is a hormone generated from adipocytes that has anti-inflammatory characteristics. It is essential for regulating insulin sensitivity. Adiponectin levels and insulin resistance are inversely correlated, according to clinical research, with patients with metabolic diseases and obese people having lower adiponectin levels [4, 12]. Mechanistic investigations have demonstrated that adiponectin improves insulin sensitivity by triggering fatty acid oxidation and activating AMP-activated protein kinase (AMPK), which counteracts the inflammatory effects of IL-6 and TNF-α [4, 13].

Adipokines including resistin and leptin, in addition to cytokines, have been linked to the pathophysiology of insulin resistance. The hormone leptin, which is mostly released by adipocytes, controls hunger and energy balance. By influencing hypothalamic signalling pathways, it can also affect insulin sensitivity [14, 15]. Another adipokine called resistin has been demonstrated to increase insulin resistance in skeletal muscle and adipose tissue by obstructing insulin signalling and glucose uptake [16, 17].

One key mechanism connecting inflammation and insulin resistance is the activation of inflammatory signalling pathways, such as c-Jun N-terminal kinase (JNK) and nuclear factor kappa B (NF-κB). Experiments have shown that activation of NF-κB causes the expression of chemokines and pro-inflammatory cytokines, which exacerbates insulin resistance and accelerates the development of metabolic diseases [1, 2]. Similarly, by phosphorylating IRS proteins and upsetting insulin signalling pathways, JNK activation leads to insulin resistance [6, 7].

Overall, the review of the literature emphasises how important it is to target inflammatory pathways to prevent and treat metabolic illnesses, as well as how important inflammation is in the pathophysiology of insulin resistance.

3. Mechanisms of insulin resistance caused by inflammation

Insulin resistance is defined by a reduced ability of target tissues, including adipose, liver, and skeletal muscle, to respond to the effects of insulin. This leads to a decrease in the absorption and metabolism of glucose. As insulin resistance develops and progresses, chronic low-grade inflammation has been shown to play a significant role. Inflammatory mediators interfere with insulin signalling pathways on several levels [1, 2].

3.1 Insulin signalling pathway dysregulation

3.1.1 IRS protein serine phosphorylation

Serine kinases, such as IκB kinase (IKK) and c-Jun N-terminal kinase (JNK), are activated by inflammatory cytokines like TNF-α and IL-6. These kinases phosphorylate insulin receptor substrate (IRS) proteins on serine residues [2, 8]. By preventing the tyrosine phosphorylation of IRS proteins, this serine phosphorylation reduces insulin sensitivity and messes with downstream insulin signalling cascades [9, 10].

3.1.2 Blocking the PI3K/Akt pathway

By phosphorylating Akt (protein kinase B), phosphatidylinositol 3-kinase (PI3K) is essential for modulating the metabolic effects of insulin. Impaired glucose uptake and glycogen production can result from direct or indirect suppression of PI3K/Akt signalling by inflammatory signalling pathways such as NF-κB and JNK [18, 19].

3.1.3 Protein kinase C (PKC) isoform activation

PKC isoforms are activated by elevated amounts of the lipid second messenger diacylglycerol (DAG), which phosphorylates insulin receptor substrate-1 (IRS-1) and inhibits insulin-stimulated glucose uptake. These actions disrupt insulin signalling [20, 21].

3.2 Mitochondrial dysfunction and oxidative stress

3.2.1 Impairment in oxidative metabolism

Prolonged inflammation can cause disturbances in the synthesis and operation of mitochondria, resulting in impaired oxidative metabolism and mitochondrial dysfunction [22]. Insulin resistance is a result of decreased mitochondrial ATP synthesis and elevated reactive oxygen species (ROS) production, which impede insulin signalling and trigger cellular stress responses [23].

3.2.2 ROS-generated inflammatory pathways

Inflammatory signalling pathways, including NF-κB and JNK, are activated by ROS produced during mitochondrial failure, aggravating inflammation and insulin resistance [24].

3.3 Lipid accretion and lipotoxicity

3.3.1 Improved lipolysis and release of free fatty acids (FFA)

TNF-α and IL-6 are examples of inflammatory cytokines that promote lipolysis in adipose tissue, which increases the amount of free fatty acids released into the bloodstream [25]. Increased circulating FFA levels encourage the buildup of lipids in non-adipose tissues such as the liver and skeletal muscle, which exacerbates insulin resistance [26].

3.3.2 Lipid intermediate formation

Overindulgence in free fatty acids (FFAs) leads to the metabolism of lipid intermediates, including DAG and ceramides, which impede insulin signalling and enhance cellular stress responses [27]. For example, ceramides activate protein phosphatase 2A (PP2A), which inhibits insulin signalling and dephosphorylates Akt [28].

3.4 Dysregulation of adipokines and inflammation of adipose tissue

3.4.1 Macrophages in adipose tissue infiltration

Adipose tissue experiences dynamic remodelling in obesity and insulin resistance, which is typified by an increase in the infiltration of immune cells and pro-inflammatory macrophages [29]. TNF-α and IL-6 are among the inflammatory cytokines secreted by these activated immune cells, which lead to both local inflammation and systemic inflammation [30].

3.4.2 Dysregulated adipokine secretion

Insulin sensitivity and energy balance are regulated by adipokines, which are secreted by adipose tissue and include adiponectin, leptin, and resistin [31]. Dysregulated insulin signalling and metabolic dysfunction might result from adipocyte malfunction and inflammatory cytokines upsetting the balance of adipokine production [32].

Comprehending the complex processes via which inflammation leads to insulin resistance offers valuable perspectives on possible treatment targets and intervention tactics.

4. Clinical implications and associations

The development and progression of several metabolic disorders, such as type 2 diabetes mellitus (T2DM), cardiovascular disease (CVD), and non-alcoholic fatty liver disease (NAFLD), are closely linked to insulin resistance, which is characterised by impaired target tissue responsiveness to insulin action. Insulin resistance has significant clinical implications. The pathophysiology of insulin resistance is largely influenced by chronic low-grade inflammation, which also contributes to the clinical symptoms and related consequences of the condition.

4.1 Correlation to T2DM (type 2 diabetes mellitus)

One of the main characteristics of type 2 diabetes is insulin resistance, which is characterised by peripheral organs such as the liver, adipose tissue, and skeletal muscle having decreased sensitivity to insulin action [1, 2].

Pro-inflammatory cytokines including TNF-α and IL-6, which are high in chronic inflammation, lead to insulin resistance and β-cell dysfunction, which in turn accelerates the development and progression of type 2 diabetes [2, 8].

High-sensitivity C-reactive protein (hs-CRP) and the risk of acquiring type 2 diabetes (T2DM) have been linked to inflammation through epidemiological research, indicating the clinical importance of inflammation-induced insulin resistance in the pathophysiology of diabetes [9, 10].

4.2 Correlation with cardiovascular disease (CVD)

Atherosclerosis, hypertension, and coronary artery disease are all made more likely in people who are insulin-resistant [33]. Insulin resistance is a major factor in determining cardiovascular risk.

By encouraging endothelial dysfunction, oxidative stress, and vascular inflammation, chronic inflammation adds to the pathophysiology of CVD by hastening the development of atherosclerosis and raising the risk of cardiovascular events [34].

The clinical relevance of inflammation-induced insulin resistance in cardiovascular health is highlighted by the greatly increased risk of cardiovascular disease (CVD) in patients with metabolic syndrome and insulin resistance [35].

4.3 Correlation with non-alcoholic fatty liver disease (NAFLD)

The emergence of NAFLD, a group of liver diseases that includes cirrhosis, non-alcoholic steatohepatitis (NASH), and simple steatosis, is directly linked to insulin resistance [36].

The aetiology of non-alcoholic fatty liver disease (NAFLD) is aided by hepatic insulin resistance, which raises hepatic glucose synthesis, *de novo* lipogenesis, and triglyceride accumulation [37].

Pro-inflammatory cytokines stimulate hepatic inflammation, fibrosis, and hepatocyte death, all of which are important factors in the development of non-alcoholic fatty liver disease (NAFLD) [38].

4.4 Clinical relevance for risk evaluation and control

Evaluation of inflammatory markers, including hs-CRP, interleukins, and adipokines, might give important information on the underlying inflammatory state and cardiovascular risk profile of insulin-resistant people [39].

It has been demonstrated that dietary changes, physical activity, and weight loss are among the lifestyle therapies that target inflammation and can enhance insulin sensitivity and lower cardiovascular risk in people with metabolic disorders [40].

Additional advantages in lowering cardiovascular risk and enhancing clinical outcomes for people with insulin resistance may come from pharmacological therapies like anti-inflammatory drugs and statins [41].

In order to reduce the burden of metabolic disorders and cardiovascular consequences, it is imperative to understand the clinical implications and connections of inflammation-induced insulin resistance. This will help with risk assessment, early detection, and focused intervention options.

5. Diagnostic tools and biomarkers

Determining the risk of the disease, directing therapeutic approaches, and gauging the effectiveness of treatment all depend on the accurate diagnosis and monitoring of inflammation-induced insulin resistance. In clinical practice and research settings, a variety of diagnostic instruments and biomarkers have been developed to measure insulin sensitivity and identify inflammation.

5.1 Inflammatory markers

5.1.1 High-sensitivity C-reactive protein (hs-CRP)

hs-CRP is a commonly used biomarker of cardiovascular risk and systemic inflammation. Insulin resistance, metabolic syndrome, and an increased risk of cardiovascular events are all linked to elevated levels of hs-CRP [42, 43].

5.1.2 Interleukins (ILs)

The pro-inflammatory cytokines IL-6, IL-1β, and IL-18 are linked to the aetiology of metabolic diseases and insulin resistance. When circulating IL levels are measured in insulin-resistant individuals, it offers valuable information about their level of inflammation and the severity of their condition [9, 10].

5.1.3 Tumour necrosis factor-alpha (TNF-α)

TNF-α is an important modulator of insulin resistance brought on by inflammation, causing IRS protein serine phosphorylation and disrupting insulin signalling. Obesity, type 2 diabetes, and other metabolic diseases are associated with elevated levels of TNF-α [3, 8].

5.2 Adipokines

5.2.1 Adiponectin

This hormone, which is produced from adipocytes, has anti-inflammatory and insulin-sensitising characteristics. Obesity, insulin resistance, and cardiovascular risk are linked to decreased adiponectin levels [4, 12].

5.2.2 Leptin

Adipocytes secrete the hormone leptin, which controls hunger and energy balance. Obesity and insulin resistance are associated with elevated leptin levels, which are indicative of leptin resistance and dysfunctional adipose tissue [14, 15].

5.3 Lipid biomarkers

5.3.1 Free fatty acids (FFAs)

By encouraging fat accumulation in non-adipose tissues and disrupting insulin signalling, elevated circulating FFAs contribute to insulin resistance. In those with metabolic diseases, measuring FFAs offers information on insulin sensitivity and lipid metabolism [26].

5.3.2 Lipid intermediates

Insulin resistance and metabolic dysfunction have been linked to ceramides, diacylglycerols (DAGs), and other lipid intermediates. Type 2 diabetes, NAFLD, and obesity are all associated with elevated levels of lipid intermediates [44].

5.4 Imaging techniques

5.4.1 Magnetic resonance imaging (MRI) and positron emission tomography (PET)

These methods provide non-invasive evaluation of metabolic activity, insulin sensitivity, and tissue-specific glucose uptake. The pathogenesis of insulin resistance and metabolic diseases can be better understood by using these imaging modalities [45].

5.4.2 Dual-energy X-ray absorptiometry (DEXA) and computed tomography (CT)

These scans are used to measure visceral adiposity and ectopic fat deposition. Insulin resistance and an elevated risk of cardiovascular disease are linked to ectopic fat deposition and abdominal obesity [46].

5.5 Functional tests

5.5.1 Hyperinsulinemic euglycemic clamp and oral glucose tolerance test (OGTT)

Both are the gold standard tests for determining insulin sensitivity and glucose tolerance, respectively. In those with insulin resistance, these functional tests offer quantitative assessments of insulin action and metabolic function [47].

5.6 Molecular and genetic biomarkers

5.6.1 Single-nucleotide polymorphisms (SNPs)

The pathophysiology of insulin resistance and metabolic diseases has been linked to genetic variants linked to genes related to inflammation, such as TNF-α and IL-6. People who are more likely to develop insulin resistance due to inflammation may benefit from genetic testing [48].

5.6.2 Gene expression profiling

This technique enables a thorough examination of the gene expression patterns linked to insulin resistance and inflammation. The development of tailored therapeutics may be aided by molecular profiling approaches, which offer insights into the molecular pathways underlying disease pathogenesis [49].

6. Therapeutic strategies

Targeting both inflammatory pathways and metabolic dysfunction is necessary for the effective therapy of inflammation-induced insulin resistance. Numerous medication and lifestyle strategies have been created to enhance insulin sensitivity, lower inflammation, and lessen the chance of related metabolic problems.

6.1 Pharmacological interventions

6.1.1 Anti-inflammatory agents

The potential of nonsteroidal anti-inflammatory medicines (NSAIDs) like aspirin and ibuprofen, as well as selective inhibitors of inflammatory pathways like TNF-α antagonists and IL-1β blockers, to reduce systemic inflammation and improve insulin sensitivity has been studied [50, 51].

6.1.2 PPAR-γ agonists

The nuclear receptor known as peroxisome proliferator-activated receptor gamma (PPAR-γ), which is involved in the control of adipogenesis and insulin sensitivity, is agonistic to thiazolidinediones (TZDs), which include pioglitazone and rosiglitazone. By regulating adipokine production and reducing the expression of inflammatory genes, TZDs enhance insulin sensitivity and decrease inflammation [52, 53].

6.1.3 AMPK activators

A major modulator of insulin sensitivity and cellular energy metabolism is AMP-activated protein kinase (AMPK). Metformin and thiazolidinediones are examples of AMPK activators that improve insulin signalling and glucose absorption in target tissues by blocking mTOR signalling and activating AMPK [54, 55].

6.1.4 SGLT2 inhibitors

In people with type 2 diabetes mellitus, sodium-glucose cotransporter 2 (SGLT2) inhibitors, such as dapagliflozin and empagliflozin, decrease renal glucose reabsorption and increase urine glucose excretion, improving glycemic control and insulin sensitivity [56, 57].

6.1.5 GLP-1 receptor agonists

GLP-1 receptor agonists (GLP-1RAs) have surfaced as promising therapeutic options, boasting potent anti-inflammatory characteristics and a wide range of clinical applications [58].

6.2 Combination therapies

6.2.1 Dual PPAR-α/γ agonists

Preclinical and clinical investigations have demonstrated the potential of combination treatments that target various metabolic pathways to improve insulin sensitivity and reduce inflammation [59, 60].

6.2.2 Multimodal interventions

Behavioural counselling, exercise, and diet combined with pharmaceutical medications may provide synergistic effects in the management of metabolic diseases and inflammation-induced insulin resistance [61, 62].

6.3 Emerging therapeutic targets

6.3.1 Microbiome modulation

There may be a connection between insulin resistance, inflammation, and the gut microbiota composition, as per emerging research. Probiotics, prebiotics, and faecal microbiota transplantation are examples of strategies that target the gut microbiome and show promise as innovative therapeutic approaches for enhancing metabolic health [63, 64].

6.3.2 Epigenetic modification

Patterns of gene expression linked to inflammation and insulin resistance are regulated by epigenetic changes, including DNA methylation and histone acetylation. Histone deacetylase inhibitors and DNA methyltransferase inhibitors are examples of epigenetic modulators that may be used as therapeutic targets [65, 66].

7. Lifestyle interventions

7.1 Dietary changes

Embracing a nutritious diet high in fruits, vegetables, whole grains, and lean meats can help lower inflammation and enhance insulin sensitivity. Low-glycemic index and

Mediterranean-style diets have been linked to better metabolic health and decreased systemic inflammation [67, 68].

7.2 Frequent exercise

Exercise is essential for lowering inflammation, encouraging weight loss, and enhancing insulin sensitivity. In those with insulin resistance, aerobic exercise and resistance training have both been demonstrated to improve glucose uptake, insulin action, and metabolic function [69, 70].

7.3 Handling weight

Insulin resistance and systemic inflammation are closely linked to obesity. Insulin sensitivity and metabolic parameters can be significantly improved by weight loss attained through calorie restriction, behavioural therapies, and bariatric surgery [71, 72].

8. Prospects for future research and directions

Progress in comprehending the intricate relationship among inflammation, insulin resistance, and metabolic dysfunction has created opportunities for novel approaches to treatment and investigation. It is highly promising that future research will clarify the molecular processes of inflammation-induced insulin resistance and find new targets for treatment, as these efforts will help to improve metabolic health and lessen the burden of related disorders.

8.1 Targeted therapies

8.1.1 Precision medicine methods

Individualised treatment plans based on genetic predispositions, inflammatory status, and metabolic profiles may enhance therapeutic efficacy and minimise side effects. Targeted therapeutics for inflammation-induced insulin resistance can be developed more easily when genomic, proteomic, and metabolomic data are integrated into clinical practice [73, 74].

8.1.2 Novel drug targets

The discovery and confirmation of new pharmacological targets related to the control of insulin signalling, metabolic homeostasis, and inflammatory pathways present promising prospects for the creation of next-generation treatments. The potential of emerging targets, like cytokine receptors, Toll-like receptors (TLRs), and inflammasomes, to reduce inflammation and enhance insulin sensitivity calls for more research [75, 76].

8.2 Metabolic crosstalk and immunometabolism

8.2.1 Immunometabolic pathways

Immunometabolism, the integration of immunological and metabolic signalling pathways, offers new perspectives on the aetiology of metabolic diseases including insulin resistance. Finding new treatment targets for inflammation-induced insulin resistance may be possible by clarifying the molecular mechanisms underlying immune cell metabolism, cytokine signalling, and metabolic reprogramming [77, 78].

8.2.2 Metabolic crosstalk

The control of systemic inflammation and insulin sensitivity is greatly influenced by communication between several metabolic organs and tissues, including adipose tissue, the liver, muscle, and the gut microbiota. Novel treatments that target metabolic crosstalk and dysregulation may be developed as a result of a better understanding of the reciprocal connections between immune cells and metabolic organs [78, 79].

8.3 Integrated omics methods

8.3.1 Multi-omics profiling

Integrating data from multiple fields, including proteomics, metabolomics, transcriptomics, and genomes, holds potential for a thorough understanding of the molecular mechanisms driving inflammation-induced insulin resistance. Network analysis and pathway modelling are two examples of systems biology techniques that can offer comprehensive insights into the pathophysiology of disease and suggest possible targets for treatment [80, 81].

8.3.2 Artificial intelligence and machine learning

Identification of predictive biomarkers, disease subtypes, and therapeutic response profiles are made possible by the use of artificial intelligence (AI) techniques and machine learning algorithms to large-scale omics datasets. The development of innovative therapeutic approaches and individualised treatment plans for inflammation-induced insulin resistance may proceed more quickly if AI-driven analytics is fully utilised [82, 83].

8.4 Behaviour interventions and lifestyle changes

8.4.1 Digital health technologies

By incorporating wearables, smartphone apps, and remote monitoring platforms with lifestyle treatments and behavioural change programmes, digital health technologies can improve patient outcomes, adherence, and engagement. Digital health platforms that enable social support networks, real-time feedback, and personalised coaching may enhance metabolic results and long-term adherence to healthy behaviours [84, 85].

8.4.2 Behavioural economics

The development of successful interventions targeted at encouraging healthy lifestyle choices and reducing the risk of inflammation-induced insulin resistance can be aided by behavioural economics insights such as choice architecture and nudge theory. Behavioural interventions that apply behavioural economics concepts—like default options, framing effects, and incentive structures—may help modify behaviour in a sustainable way and enhance metabolic health outcomes [86, 87].

9. Conclusion

Insulin resistance brought on by inflammation is a complicated metabolic disease with wide-ranging effects on human health. Despite tremendous advancements in our comprehension of the underlying pathophysiological pathways, effective therapeutic approaches for insulin resistance caused by inflammation are still unattainable.

In order to fully understand the complex interactions between inflammation and insulin signalling pathways, a multidisciplinary approach integrating knowledge from immunology, metabolism, genetics, and systems biology is essential going ahead. Personalised treatment plans, lifestyle changes, and targeted pharmaceutical interventions have the potential to enhance metabolic health and lessen the impact of comorbidities linked to inflammation-induced insulin resistance.

Furthermore, improving our knowledge of inflammation-induced insulin resistance and integrating scientific findings into clinical practice depend on ongoing research efforts focused on identifying novel therapeutic targets, clarifying the molecular mechanisms underlying disease pathogenesis, and creating cutting-edge diagnostic tools and biomarkers.

We can overcome the obstacles presented by inflammation-induced insulin resistance and open the door to the creation of efficient preventive and treatment plans that enhance the lives of those impacted by this common and crippling metabolic illness by adopting a collaborative and interdisciplinary research paradigm.

Author details

Anchala Kumari
Arontier, Seoul, South Korea

*Address all correspondence to: anchala.choudhary27@gmail.com

References

[1] Hotamisligil GS. Inflammation and metabolic disorders. Nature. 2006;**444**(7121):860-867

[2] Shoelson SE, Lee J, Goldfine AB. Inflammation and insulin resistance. Journal of Clinical Investigation. 2006;**116**(7):1793-1801

[3] Pickup JC, Crook MA, Ismail IH. TNF-α, interleukin-1, and insulin resistance in obesity. Biochemical Society Transactions. 2000;**28**(2):522-526

[4] Yamauchi T, Kamon J, Waki H, Terauchi Y, Kubota N, Hara K, et al. The fat-derived hormone adiponectin reverses insulin resistance associated with both lipoatrophy and obesity. Nature Medicine. 2001;**7**(8):941-946

[5] Hotamisligil GS. Endoplasmic reticulum stress and the inflammatory basis of metabolic disease. Cell. 2010;**140**(6):900-917

[6] Hirosumi J, Tuncman G, Chang L, Görgün CZ, Uysal KT, Maeda K, et al. A central role for JNK in obesity and insulin resistance. Nature. 2002;**420**(6913):333-336

[7] Gual P, Le Marchand-Brustel Y, Tanti JF. Positive and negative regulation of insulin signaling through IRS-1 phosphorylation. Biochimie. 2007;**89**(6-7):1-9

[8] Hotamisligil GS. Mechanisms of TNF-alpha-induced insulin resistance. Experimental and Clinical Endocrinology & Diabetes. 1999;**107**(2):119-125

[9] Pedersen BK, Febbraio MA. Muscle as an endocrine organ: Focus on muscle-derived interleukin-6. Physiological Reviews. 2008;**88**(4): 1379-1406

[10] Carey AL, Steinberg GR, Macaulay SL, Thomas WG, Holmes AG, Ramm G, et al. Interleukin-6 increases insulin-stimulated glucose disposal in humans and glucose uptake and fatty acid oxidation in vitro via AMP-activated protein kinase. Diabetes. 2006;**55**(10):2688-2697

[11] Senn JJ, Klover PJ, Nowak IA, Mooney RA. Interleukin-6 induces cellular insulin resistance in hepatocytes. Diabetes. 2002;**51**(12):3391-3399

[12] Arita Y, Kihara S, Ouchi N, Takahashi M, Maeda K, Miyagawa J, et al. Paradoxical decrease of an adipose-specific protein, adiponectin, in obesity. Biochemical and Biophysical Research Communications. 1999;**257**(1):79-83

[13] Berg AH, Combs TP, Du X, Brownlee M, Scherer PE. The adipocyte-secreted protein Acrp30 enhances hepatic insulin action. Nature Medicine. 2001;**7**(8):947-953

[14] Maffei M, Halaas J, Ravussin E, Pratley RE, Lee GH, Zhang Y, et al. Leptin levels in human and rodent: Measurement of plasma leptin and Ob RNA in obese and weight-reduced subjects. Nature Medicine. 1995;**1**(11):1155-1161

[15] Mantzoros CS, Magkos F, Brinkoetter M, Sienkiewicz E, Dardeno TA, Kim SY, et al. Leptin in human physiology and pathophysiology. American Journal of Physiology. Endocrinology and Metabolism. 2011;**301**(4):E567-E584

[16] Steppan CM, Bailey ST, Bhat S, Brown EJ, Banerjee RR, Wright CM, et al. The hormone resistin links obesity to diabetes. Nature. 2001;**409**(6818):307-312

[17] Satoh H, Nguyen MT, Miles PD, Imamura T, Usui I, Olefsky JM, et al. Adenovirus-mediated chronic "hyper-resistinemia" leads to in vivo insulin resistance in normal rats. Journal of Clinical Investigation. 2004;**114**(2):224-231

[18] Ramasubbu K, Devi RV. Impairment of insulin signaling pathway PI3K/Akt/mTOR and insulin resistance induced AGEs on diabetes mellitus and neurodegenerative diseases: A perspective review. Molecular and Cellular Biochemistry. 2023;**478**(6):1307-1324

[19] ElMahdy MK, Zaki MO, Al-Karmalawy AA, Abdo W, Alnasser SM, Antar SA. Glimepiride ameliorates renal toxicity induced by cadmium in mice: Modulation of Jun N terminal kinase (JNK)/nuclear factor kappa B (NF-κB) and phosphatidylinositol 3-kinases (PI3K)/protein kinase (AKT) pathways. Life Sciences. 2022;**311**:121184

[20] Kolczynska K, Loza-Valdes A, Hawro I, Sumara G. Diacylglycerol-evoked activation of PKC and PKD isoforms in regulation of glucose and lipid metabolism: A review. Lipids in Health and Disease. 2020;**19**:1-5

[21] Turban S, Hajduch E. Protein kinase C isoforms: Mediators of reactive lipid metabolites in the development of insulin resistance. FEBS Letters. 2011;**585**(2):269-274

[22] Prasun P. Mitochondrial dysfunction in metabolic syndrome. Biochimica et Biophysica Acta (BBA) - Molecular Basis of Disease. 2020;**1866**(10):165838

[23] Ayer A, Fazakerley DJ, James DE, Stocker R. The role of mitochondrial reactive oxygen species in insulin resistance. Free Radical Biology and Medicine. 2022;**179**:339-362

[24] Choudhury S, Ghosh S, Gupta P, Mukherjee S, Chattopadhyay S. Inflammation-induced ROS generation causes pancreatic cell death through modulation of Nrf2/NF-κB and SAPK/JNK pathway. Free Radical Research. 2015;**49**(11):1371-1383

[25] Kojta I, Chacińska M, Błachnio-Zabielska A. Obesity, bioactive lipids, and adipose tissue inflammation in insulin resistance. Nutrients. 2020;**12**(5):1305

[26] Ahmed B, Sultana R, Greene MW. Adipose tissue and insulin resistance in obese. Biomedicine and Pharmacotherapy. 2021;**137**:111315

[27] Sinha S, Haque M. Obesity, diabetes mellitus, and vascular impediment as consequences of excess processed food consumption. Cureus. 2022;**14**(9):1-24

[28] Bharath LP, Ruan T, Li Y, Ravindran A, Wan X, Nhan JK, et al. Ceramide-initiated protein phosphatase 2A activation contributes to arterial dysfunction in vivo. Diabetes. 2015;**64**(11):3914-3926

[29] Vieira-Potter VJ. Inflammation and macrophage modulation in adipose tissues. Cellular Microbiology. 2014;**16**(10):1484-1492

[30] Wang T, He C. TNF-α and IL-6: The link between immune and bone system. Current Drug Targets. 2020;**21**(3):213-227

[31] Ahima RS, Lazar MA. Adipokines and the peripheral and neural control of energy balance. Molecular Endocrinology. 2008;**22**(5):1023-1031

[32] Lafontan M. Adipose tissue and adipocyte dysregulation. Diabetes & Metabolism. 2014;**40**(1):16-28

[33] DeFronzo RA, Ferrannini E. Insulin resistance: A multifaceted syndrome responsible for NIDDM, obesity, hypertension, dyslipidemia, and atherosclerotic cardiovascular disease. Diabetes Care. 1991;**14**(3):173-194

[34] Mason JC, Libby P. Cardiovascular disease in patients with chronic inflammation: Mechanisms underlying premature cardiovascular events in rheumatologic conditions. European Heart Journal. 2015;**36**(8):482-489

[35] Romeo GR, Lee J, Shoelson SE. Metabolic syndrome, insulin resistance, and roles of inflammation–mechanisms and therapeutic targets. Arteriosclerosis, Thrombosis, and Vascular Biology. 2012;**32**(8):1771-1776

[36] Liu Q, Bengmark S, Qu S. The role of hepatic fat accumulation in pathogenesis of non-alcoholic fatty liver disease (NAFLD). Lipids in Health and Disease. 2010;**9**:1-9

[37] Mu W, Cheng XF, Liu Y, Lv QZ, Liu GL, Zhang JG, et al. Potential nexus of non-alcoholic fatty liver disease and type 2 diabetes mellitus: Insulin resistance between hepatic and peripheral tissues. Frontiers in Pharmacology. 2019;**9**:1566

[38] Duan Y, Pan X, Luo J, Xiao X, Li J, Bestman PL, et al. Association of inflammatory cytokines with non-alcoholic fatty liver disease. Frontiers in Immunology. 2022;**13**:880298

[39] Sutherland JP, McKinley B, Eckel RH. The metabolic syndrome and inflammation. Metabolic Syndrome and Related Disorders. 2004;**2**(2):82-104

[40] Andersen CJ, Fernandez ML. Dietary strategies to reduce metabolic syndrome. Reviews in Endocrine and Metabolic Disorders. 2013;**14**:241-254

[41] Ruscica M, Corsini A, Ferri N, Banach M, Sirtori CR. Clinical approach to the inflammatory etiology of cardiovascular diseases. Pharmacological Research. 2020;**159**:104916

[42] Ridker PM. Clinical application of C-reactive protein for cardiovascular disease detection and prevention. Circulation. 2003;**107**(3):363-369

[43] Pradhan AD, Manson JE, Rifai N, Buring JE, Ridker PM. C-reactive protein, interleukin 6, and risk of developing type 2 diabetes mellitus. JAMA. 2001;**286**(3):327-334

[44] Kitessa SM, Abeywardena MY. Lipid-induced insulin resistance in skeletal muscle: The chase for the culprit goes from total intramuscular fat to lipid intermediates, and finally to species of lipid intermediates. Nutrients. 2016;**8**(8):466

[45] Johansson E, Lubberink M, Heurling K, Eriksson JW, Skrtic S, Ahlström H, et al. Whole-body imaging of tissue-specific insulin sensitivity and body composition by using an integrated PET/MR system: A feasibility study. Radiology. 2018;**286**(1):271-278

[46] Kaul S, Rothney MP, Peters DM, Wacker WK, Davis CE, Shapiro MD, et al. Dual-energy X-ray absorptiometry for quantification of visceral fat. Obesity. Jun 2012;**20**(6):1313-1318

[47] Pratt-Phillips SE, Geor RJ, McCutcheon LJ. Comparison among the euglycemic-hyperinsulinemic clamp, insulin-modified frequently sampled intravenous glucose tolerance test, and oral glucose tolerance test for assessment of insulin sensitivity in healthy

Standardbreds. American Journal of Veterinary Research. 2015;**76**(1):84-91

[48] Malodobra M, Pilecka A, Gworys B, Adamiec R. Single nucleotide polymorphisms within functional regions of genes implicated in insulin action and association with the insulin resistant phenotype. Molecular and Cellular Biochemistry. 2011;**349**:187-193

[49] Konstantopoulos N, Foletta VC, Segal DH, Shields KA, Sanigorski A, Windmill K, et al. A gene expression signature for insulin resistance. Physiological Genomics. 2011;**43**(3):110-120

[50] Ridker PM, Lüscher TF. Anti-inflammatory therapies for cardiovascular disease. European Heart Journal. 2014;**35**(27):1782-1791

[51] Gómez-García A, Hernández-Campos ME. An update on the use of TNF-α inhibitors in the treatment of psoriasis. Drug Design, Development and Therapy. 2016;**10**:1581-1591

[52] Yki-Järvinen H. Thiazolidinediones. New England Journal of Medicine. 2004;**351**(11):1106-1118

[53] Zinman B, Wanner C, Lachin JM, Fitchett D, Bluhmki E, Hantel S, et al. Empagliflozin, cardiovascular outcomes, and mortality in type 2 diabetes. New England Journal of Medicine. 2015;**373**(22):2117-2128

[54] Hardie DG. AMPK—Sensing energy while talking to other signaling pathways. Cell Metabolism. 2014;**20**(6):939-952

[55] Viollet B, Guigas B, Sanz Garcia N, Leclerc J, Foretz M, Andreelli F. Cellular and molecular mechanisms of metformin: An overview. Clinical Science. 2012;**122**(6):253-270

[56] DeFronzo RA, Norton L, Abdul-Ghani M. Renal, metabolic and cardiovascular considerations of SGLT2 inhibition. Nature Reviews Nephrology. 2017;**13**(1):11-26

[57] Abdul-Ghani M, Del Prato S, Chilton R, DeFronzo RA. SGLT2 inhibitors and cardiovascular risk: Lessons learned from the EMPA-REG OUTCOME Study. Diabetes Care. 2016;**39**(5):717-725

[58] Alharbi SH. Anti-inflammatory role of glucagon-like peptide 1 receptor agonists and its clinical implications. Therapeutic Advances in Endocrinology and Metabolism. 2024;**15**:20420188231222367

[59] Marx N, Duez H. Peroxisome proliferator-activated receptors and atherogenesis: Regulators of gene expression in vascular cells. Circulation Research. 2007;**100**(6):803-817

[60] Fougerat A, Gayral S, Gourdy P, Schambourg A. Dual PPARα/γ agonists: Promising new targets in the treatment of type 2 diabetes and associated complications. Current Opinion in Pharmacology. 2019;**49**:106-115

[61] Look AHEAD Research Group. Reduction in weight and cardiovascular disease risk factors in individuals with type 2 diabetes: One-year results of the Look AHEAD trial. Diabetes Care. 2007;**30**(6):1374-1383

[62] Knowler WC, Barrett-Connor E, Fowler SE, Hamman RF, Lachin JM, Walker EA, et al. Reduction in the incidence of type 2 diabetes with lifestyle intervention or metformin. New England Journal of Medicine. 2002;**346**(6):393-403

[63] Cani PD, Amar J, Iglesias MA, Poggi M, Knauf C, Bastelica D, et al.

Metabolic endotoxemia initiates obesity and insulin resistance. Diabetes. 2007;**56**(7):1761-1772

[64] Vrieze A, Van Nood E, Holleman F, Salojärvi J, Kootte RS, Bartelsman JFWM, et al. Transfer of intestinal microbiota from lean donors increases insulin sensitivity in individuals with metabolic syndrome. Gastroenterology. 2012;**143**(4):913-916.e7

[65] Ling C, Rönn T. Epigenetics in human obesity and type 2 diabetes. Cell Metabolism. 2019;**29**(5):1028-1044

[66] Barres R, Zierath JR. DNA methylation in metabolic disorders. American Journal of Clinical Nutrition. 2011;**93**(4):897S-900S

[67] Esposito K, Marfella R, Ciotola M, Di Palo C, Giugliano F, Giugliano G, et al. Effect of a Mediterranean-style diet on endothelial dysfunction and markers of vascular inflammation in the metabolic syndrome: A randomized trial. JAMA. 2004;**292**(12):1440-1446

[68] Jenkins DJA, Kendall CWC, Augustin LSA, Franceschi S, Hamidi M, Marchie A, et al. Glycemic index: Overview of implications in health and disease. American Journal of Clinical Nutrition. 2002;**76**(1):266S-273S

[69] Hawley JA, Lessard SJ. Exercise training-induced improvements in insulin action. Acta Physiologica. 2008;**192**(1):127-135

[70] Church TS, Blair SN, Cocreham S, Johannsen N, Johnson W, Kramer K, et al. Effects of aerobic and resistance training on hemoglobin A1c levels in patients with type 2 diabetes. JAMA. 2010;**304**(20):2253-2262

[71] Lean MEJ, Malkova D. Altered gut and adipose tissue hormones in overweight and obese individuals: Cause or consequence? International Journal of Obesity. 2016;**40**(4):622-632

[72] Pi-Sunyer FX. The epidemiology of central fat distribution in relation to disease. Nutrition Reviews. 2009;**67**(suppl_2):S81-S84

[73] Collins FS, Varmus H. A new initiative on precision medicine. New England Journal of Medicine. 2015;**372**(9):793-795

[74] Khera AV, Chaffin M, Aragam KG, Haas ME, Roselli C, Choi SH, et al. Genome-wide polygenic scores for common diseases identify individuals with risk equivalent to monogenic mutations. Nature Genetics. 2018;**50**(9):1219-1224

[75] Swanson KV, Deng M, Ting JPY. The NLRP3 inflammasome: Molecular activation and regulation to therapeutics. Nature Reviews Immunology. 2019;**19**(8):477-489

[76] O'Neill LAJ, Netea MG. BCG-induced trained immunity: Can it offer protection against COVID-19? Nature Reviews Immunology. 2020;**20**(6):335-337

[77] Odegaard JI, Chawla A. Connecting type 1 and type 2 diabetes through innate immunity. Cold Spring Harbor Perspectives in Medicine. 2013;**3**(3):a007724

[78] Hotamisligil GS. Inflammation, metaflammation and immunometabolic disorders. Nature. 2017;**542**(7640):177-185

[79] Tilg H, Moschen AR. Microbiota and diabetes: An evolving relationship. Gut. 2014;**63**(9):1513-1521

[80] Hasin Y, Seldin M, Lusis A. Multi-omics approaches to disease. Genome Biology. 2017;**18**(1):83

[81] Mardinoglu A, Nielsen J. Systems medicine and metabolic modelling. Journal of Internal Medicine. 2015;**278**(6):587-596

[82] Obermeyer Z, Emanuel EJ. Predicting the future—Big data, machine learning, and clinical medicine. New England Journal of Medicine. 2016;**375**(13):1216-1219

[83] Topol EJ. High-performance medicine: The convergence of human and artificial intelligence. Nature Medicine. 2019;**25**(1):44-56

[84] Huckvale K, Morrison C, Ouyang J, Ghaghda A, Car J. The evolution of mobile apps for asthma: An updated systematic assessment of content and tools. BMC Medicine. 2019;**17**(1):58

[85] Patel MS, Volpp KG, Rosin R, Bellamy SL, Small DS, Heuer J, et al. A randomized trial of social comparison feedback and financial incentives to increase physical activity. American Journal of Health Promotion. 2018;**32**(4):935-942

[86] Thaler RH, Sunstein CR. Nudge: Improving Decisions about Health, Wealth, and Happiness. Penguin; 24 Feb 2009

[87] Loewenstein G, Brennan T, Volpp KG. Asymmetric paternalism to improve health behaviors. JAMA. 2007;**298**(20):2415-2417